Recombinant FSH
(Puregon)

Preclinical and Clinical Experience

STUDIES IN PROFERTILITY SERIES

VOLUME 5

Recombinant FSH
(Puregon)

Preclinical and Clinical Experience

**EDITED BY H. J. OUT
AND H. J. T. COELINGH BENNINK**

*The publication of this book has been made possible
by an educational grant from NV Organon*

The Parthenon Publishing Group
International Publishers in Medicine, Science & Technology

Published in the USA by
The Parthenon Publishing Group Inc.
One Blue Hill Plaza
PO Box 1564, Pearl River,
New York 10965, USA

Published in the UK by
The Parthenon Publishing Group Limited
Casterton Hall, Carnforth,
Lancs LA6 2LA, UK

Copyright © 1996 Parthenon Publishing Group

Library of Congress Cataloging-in-Publication Data
Recombinant FSH (Puregon) : preclinical and clinical experience /
  edited by H.J. Out and H.J.T Coelingh Bennink.
    p.   cm. — (Studies in profertility series ; v. 5)
  Includes bibliographical references and index.
  ISBN 1-85070-746-4
  1. Recombinant FSH—Therapeutic use—Testing. 2. Recombinant FSH—
  Testing. 3. Infertility—Chemotherapy—Evaluation. I. Out, H.J. (Henk Jan)
  II. Coelingh Bennink, Herman Jan Tymen, 1943– . III. Series.
  [DNLM: 1. Infertility—therapy. 2. FSH—therapeutic use.
  3. Recombinant Proteins—therapeutic use. W1 ST936F v.5 1996 / WP
  570 R311 1996]
  RM291.2.F64R43   1996
  615'.766—dc20
  DNLM/DLC
  for Library of Congress   96-20463
                                                                              CIP

British Library Cataloguing in Publication Data
Recombinant FSH (Puregon): preclinical and clinical experience. – (Studies in
  profertility series; v. 5)
  1. Follicle-stimulating hormone – Physiological effect 2. Infertility –
  Effect of drugs on 3. Reproduction – Effect of drugs on
  I. Out, Henk Jan II. Coelingh Bennink, H.J.T.
  618.1'78'061

ISBN 1-85070-746-4

First published 1996

*No part of this book may be reproduced
in any form without permission from the publishers except for the
quotation of brief passages for the purposes of review.*

Typeset by Martin Lister Publishing Services, Carnforth, Lancs
Printed and bound by Butler & Tanner Ltd., London and Frome, UK

Contents

List of principal contributors	ix
Preface	xi
Acknowledgements	xii

Section I Preclinical aspects

1 Comparative *in vitro* and *in vivo* studies on the biological characteristics of recombinant human follicle-stimulating hormone
B.M.J.L. Mannaerts, R. de Leeuw, J. Geelen, A. Van Ravestein, P. Van Wezenbeek, A. Schuurs and H. Kloosterboer
From *Endocrinology*, **129** (5) 2623–2630 (1991). Copyright 1991 The Endocrine Society, reproduced with permission ... 3

2 Effects of recombinant human follicle stimulating hormone on cultured human granulosa cells: comparison with urinary gonadotrophins and actions in preovulatory follicles
H.D. Mason, B.M.J.L. Mannaerts, R. de Leeuw, D.S. Willis and S. Franks
From *Human Reproduction*, **8** (11) 1823–1827 (1993). Copyright Oxford University Press, reproduced with permission ... 23

3 Circulating bioactive and immunoreactive recombinant human follicle stimulating hormone (Org 32489) after administration to gonadotropin-deficient subjects
T. Matikainen, R. de Leeuw, B.M.J.L. Mannaerts and I. Huhtaniemi
From *Fertility and Sterility*, **61** (1) 62–69 (1994). Reproduced with permission of the publisher, the American Society for Reproductive Medicine (formerly The American Fertility Society) ... 35

4 Folliculogenesis in hypophysectomized rats after treatment with recombinant human follicle-stimulating hormone
B.M.J.L. Mannaerts, J. Uilenbroek, P. Schot and R. de Leeuw
From *Biology of Reproduction*, **51**, 72–81 (1994). Reproduced with permission of The Society for the Study of Reproduction ... 49

Section II Clinical aspects

5 First established pregnancy and birth after ovarian stimulation with recombinant human follicle stimulating hormone (Org 32489) 69
P. Devroey, B.M.J.L. Mannaerts, J. Smitz, H.J.T. Coelingh Bennink and A. Van Steirteghem
From *Human Reproduction*, **8** (6) 863–865 (1993). Copyright Oxford University Press, reproduced with permission

6 Human recombinant follicle-stimulating hormone induces growth of preovulatory follicles without concomitant increase in androgen and estrogen biosynthesis in a woman with isolated gonadotropin deficiency 75
D.C. Schoot, H.J.T. Coelingh Bennink, B.M.J.L. Mannaerts, S.W.J. Lamberts, P. Bouchard and B.C.J.M. Fauser
From *Journal of Clinical Endocrinology and Metabolism*, **74** (6) 1471–1473 (1992). Copyright 1992 The Endocrine Society, reproduced with permission

7 Single-dose pharmacokinetics and pharmocodynamics of recombinant human follicle-stimulating hormone (Org 32489) in gonadotropin-deficient volunteers 85
B.M.J.L. Mannaerts, Z. Shoham, D. Schoot, P. Bouchard, J. Harlin, B. Fauser, H. Jacobs, F. Rombout and H.J.T. Coelingh Bennink
From *Fertility and Sterility*, **59** (1) 108–114 (1993). Reproduced with permission of the publisher, the American Society for Reproductive Medicine (formerly The American Fertility Society)

8 Clinical outcome of a pilot efficacy study on recombinant human follicle-stimulating hormone (Org 32489) combined with various gonadotrophin-releasing hormone agonist regimens 99
P. Devroey, B.M.J.L. Mannaerts, J. Smitz, H.J.T. Coelingh Bennink and A. Van Steirteghem
From *Human Reproduction*, **9** (6) 1064–1069 (1994). Copyright Oxford University Press, reproduced with permission

9 Recombinant human follicle-stimulating hormone and ovarian response in gonadotrophin-deficient women 115
D.C. Schoot, J. Harlin, Z. Shoham, B.M.J.L. Mannaerts, N. Lahlou, P. Bouchard, H.J.T. Coelingh Bennink and B.C.J.M. Fauser
From *Human Reproduction*, **9** (7) 1237–1242 (1994). Copyright Oxford University Press, reproduced with permission

10	First established pregnancy and birth after induction of ovulation with recombinant human follicle-stimulating hormone in polycystic ovary syndrome H.J.H.M. van Dessel, P.F.J. Donderwinkel, H.J.T. Coelingh Bennink and B.C.J.M. Fauser From *Human Reproduction*, **9** (1) 55–56 (1994). Copyright Oxford University Press, reproduced with permission	131
11	Recombinant human follicle-stimulating hormone and human chorionic gonadotropin for induction of spermatogenesis in a hypogonadotropic male S. Kliesch, H.M. Behre and E. Nieschlag From *Fertility and Sterility*, **63** (6) 1326–1328 (1995). Reproduced with permission of the publisher, the American Society for Reproductive Medicine (formerly The American Fertility Society)	137
12	Efficacy and safety of recombinant follicle stimulating hormone (Puregon®) in infertile women pituitary-suppressed with triptorelin undergoing in-vitro fertilization: a prospective, randomized, assessor-blind, multicentre trial B. Hedon, H.J. Out, J.N. Hugues, B. Camier, J. Cohen, P. Lopes, J.R. Zorn, B. van der Heijden and H.J.T. Coelingh Bennink From *Human Reproduction*, **10** (12) 3102–3106 (1995). Copyright Oxford University Press, reproduced with permission	143
13	A prospective, randomized, assessor-blind, multicentre study comparing recombinant and urinary follicle stimulating hormone (Puregon versus Metrodin) in in-vitro fertilization H.J. Out, B.M.J.L. Mannaerts, S.G.A.J. Driessen and H.J.T. Coelingh Bennink From *Human Reproduction*, **10** (10) 2534–2540 (1995). Copyright Oxford University Press, reproduced with permission	157
	Index	175

List of principal contributors

H.J.T. Coelingh Bennink
Section Reproductive Medicine
Medical Research and
 Development Unit
NV Organon
PO Box 20
5340 BH Oss
The Netherlands

H.J.H.M. van Dessel
Dijkzigt Academic Hospital
Room H 890
Dr. Molewaterplein 40
3015 GD Rotterdam
The Netherlands

P. Devroey
Center for Reproductive Medicine
Free University of Brussels
Laarbeeklaan 101
B-1090 Brussels
Belgium

B.C.J.M. Fauser
Section of Reproductive
 Endocrinology and Infertility
Department of Obstetrics and
 Gynecology
Dijkzigt University Hospital
Dr. Molewaterplein 40
3015 GD Rotterdam
The Netherlands

S. Franks
Department of Obstetrics and
 Gynaecology
Imperial College of Science
 Technology and Medicine
St Mary's Hospital Medical School
London W2 1PG
UK

I. Huhtaniemi
Department of Physiology
University of Turku
Kiinamyllynkatu 10
FIN-20520 Turku
Finland

B.M.J.L. Mannaerts
Section Reproductive Medicine
Medical Research and
 Development Unit
NV Organon
PO Box 20
5340 BH Oss
The Netherlands

E. Nieschlag
Institute of Reproductive
 Medicine
Steinfurter Straße 107
D-48149 Münster
Germany

H.J. Out
Section Reproductive Medicine
Medical Research and
 Development Unit
NV Organon
PO Box 20
5340 BH Oss
The Netherlands

Preface

The 50-year history of gonadotrophin therapy in the induction of ovulation is characterized by the source of the various preparations used. In the 1930s, after the discovery was first made that gonadal function was controlled by gonadotrophins, agents were extracted from pregnant mares. Their therapeutic effects were poor, and, as a result, science switched its attention to human sources, first the pituitary and, very soon after, the urine of postmenopausal women.

It was this latter source which would characterize gonadotrophin therapy from the early 1960s onwards; at that time, Lunenfeld and colleagues, working with a urinary preparation of hMG, had reported the first successful induction of ovulation followed by pregnancy in hypogonadotrophic anovulatory women. These original preparations of hMG were of only 5% purity. Not only were the batches produced of extraordinary variance in activity, but production was burdensome and subject to the vagaries of human supply. In recent years, increasing worldwide demand for urinary gonadotrophins has necessitated enormous urine collection programmes, but these have still been unable to cope with demands.

Although in 1995 Organon made 3.5 million visits for urine collection, it has long been clear to the company that the future of gonadotrophin therapy could not lie in urinary sources. Recombinant DNA sources would allow the large-scale production of a preparation which is almost (99%) totally pure, and which would meet the ever-increasing demand of those treating infertility by assisted conception methods. Organon developed its recombinant FSH Puregon in the search for a more efficient source with greater purity and batch-to-batch consistency.

The studies published in this volume record the preclinical and clinical development of Puregon. The papers are all selected from peer-reviewed journals and highlight the pathways taken to achieve what now signals a new age in gonadotrophin therapy. We hope that readers will enjoy the texts and benefit from the data presented.

NV Organon *Henk J. Out*
Oss *Herjan J.T. Coelingh Bennink*
The Netherlands

Acknowledgements

The Editors and Publisher would like to acknowledge with thanks the following permissions that have kindly been granted for the use of material in this publication.

The Endocrine Society for the papers: Mannaerts, B. *et al.* (1991). *Endocrinology*, **129** (5), 2623–2630 and Schoot, D.C. *et al.* (1992). *Journal of Clinical Endocrinology and Metabolism*, **74** (6), 1471–1473.

Oxford University Press for the papers: Mason, H.D. *et al.* (1993). *Human Reproduction*, **8** (11), 1823–1827, Devroey, P. *et al.* (1993). *Human Reproduction*, **8** (6), 863–865, Devroey, P. *et al.* (1994). *Human Reproduction*, **9** (6), 1064–1069, Schoot, D.C. *et al.* (1994). *Human Reproduction*, **9** (7), 1237–1242, Van Dessel, H.J.H.M. *et al.* (1994). *Human Reproduction*, **9** (1), 55–56, Hedon, B. *et al.* (1995). *Human Reproduction*, **10** (12), 3102–3106 and Out, H.J. *et al.* (1995). *Human Reproduction*, **10** (10), 2534–2540.

The Society for the Study of Reproduction for the paper: Mannaerts, B. *et al.* (1994). *Biology of Reproduction*, **51**, 72–81.

The American Society for Reproductive Medicine for the papers: Matikainen, T. *et al.* (1994). *Fertility and Sterility*, **61** (1), 62–69, Mannaerts, B. *et al.* (1993). *Fertility and Sterility*, **59** (1), 108–114 and Kliesch, S., Behre, H.M. and Nieschlag, E. (1995). *Fertility and Sterility*, **63** (6), 1326–1328.

Section I

Preclinical aspects

1

Comparative *in vitro* and *in vivo* studies on the biological characteristics of recombinant human follicle-stimulating hormone

B.M.J.L. Mannaerts, R. de Leeuw, J. Geelen, A. Van Ravestein,
P. Van Wezenbeek, A. Schuurs and H. Kloosterboer

Scientific Development Group, NV Organon,
5340 BH Oss, The Netherlands

ABSTRACT

The in vitro *and* in vivo *activities of recombinant human FSH (recFSH) produced by a Chinese hamster ovary cell line were studied and compared with those of natural FSH preparations. The specific FSH activities of recFSH established by immunoassay and* in vivo *bioassay were greater than 10,000 IU/mg protein and considerably higher than the activities of tested urinary FSH references, while the* in vivo *bio/immuno ratios of these preparations were not significantly different. Compared to a highly purified pituitary standard (IS 83/575), recFSH had a comparable high specific* in vivo *bioactivity, but the specific immunoreactivity of IS 83/575 was about 2 times lower.*

In receptor displacement and in vitro *bioassay studies recFSH provided dose-response curves parallel to those of pituitary and urinary FSH references. When equal amounts of immunoreactive FSH were tested, recFSH and urinary and pituitary FSH displayed comparable activities in both assays. The* in vitro *bioactivity of recFSH could be neutralized effectively by each of three monoclonal antibodies raised against recFSH (α-specific), urinary FSH (β-specific), and pituitary FSH αβ-specific), respectively. Moreover, 50% inhibition of comparable responses induced by recFSH, urinary "pure" FSH or pituitary FSH was established by the same amount of monoclonal antibody. These results support the structural and functional similarity of recFSH and natural*

This paper was first published in *Endocrinology,* **129** (5), 2623–2630 (1991).
Copyright 1991 The Endocrine Society, reproduced by permission

FSH. To test whether recFSH is capable of inducing LH-specific biological responses, the in vitro *induction of testosterone production in mouse Leydig cells was assessed. At least 16 IU recFSH/ml incubate were needed to increase testosterone production, indicating that the intrinsic LH bioactivity of recFSH is negligible (<0.025 mIU LH/IU FSH). The* in vivo *efficacy of recFSH was examined by treating immature female hypophysectomized rats during 4 days with recFSH only or with recFSH supplemented with hCG. RecFSH only treatment increased ovarian weight and aromatase activity in a dose-dependent manner. When recFSH dosages providing submaximal responses were supplemented with 1 IU hCG, both ovarian weight and aromatase activity were largely augmented. Neither recFSH nor urinary pure FSH, administered in a high dose was able to increase plasma estradiol levels, while ovarian weight and aromatase activity were increased to the same extent. However, when recFSH was supplemented with only 0.1 IU hCG, a 3-fold increase in median plasma estradiol levels was obtained. These findings support the two-cell two-gonadotropin theory, holding that both FSH and LH are required for estrogen biosynthesis, but also reveal that only very small amounts of LH activity are sufficient to increase estrogen secretion up to measurable plasma levels. The increases in ovarian weight, aromatase activity, and plasma estradiol induced by recFSH supplemented with 1 and 10 IU hCG were comparable to those induced by two human menopausal gonadotropin references. In conclusion, the present study demonstrates that the* in vitro *and* in vivo *biological characteristics of recFSH are indistinguishable from those of FSH isolated from natural sources.*

INTRODUCTION

FSH produced by the anterior pituitary gland plays a pivotal role in female and male reproduction by stimulating gonadal differentiation and maturation via its regulatory action on the Sertoli cell in the testis and the granulosa cell in the ovary. The mechanism of FSH action includes binding to FSH-specific plasma membrane receptors and subsequent activation of the adenylate cyclase system, resulting in the *de novo* synthesis of steroidogenic enzymes and various paracrine and endocrine factors (1,2).

In granulosa cells, FSH enhances the synthesis of aromatase cytochrome P450, resulting in an increased conversion of androgens to estrogens. Since aromatase substrate, mainly androstenedione, is produced in the thecal cell under the influence of LH, both FSH and LH are thought to be essential for estrogen biosynthesis (2, 3). The first evidence for this so-called two-cell two-gonadotropin concept was obtained several decades ago using immature hypophysectomized rats and highly purified gonadotropins (4–6). More recently, it has been suggested to re-examine the two-cell theory (7), since ovarian estradiol biosynthesis in hypogonadotropic subjects is equally well stimulated by human "pure" FSH as by human menopausal gonadotropins (hMG) containing an equal ratio of FSH to LH activity (8–10).

While natural human FSH preparations may still contain small amounts of contaminating hormones such as LH, recombinant human FSH (recFSH) is guaranteed to be free from such hormones. RecFSH has been produced by a Chinese hamster ovary (CHO) cell line transfected by the genes encoding human FSH (11). Carbohydrate structure analysis has demonstrated a close resemblance between the recombinant and the natural FSH glycans (12). Moreover, recFSH appeared to have the same charge heterogeneity as natural FSH (13). In the present study the *in vitro* and *in vivo* biological properties of recFSH were investigated and compared with those of natural human FSH. For this purpose, receptor displacement and *in vitro* bioassay studies were performed. The *in vivo* efficacy of recFSH alone or in combination with hCG was tested in immature hypophysectomized rats by measuring increases in ovarian weight, ovarian aromatase activity, and plasma estradiol levels.

MATERIALS AND METHODS

CHO cell line

Stable transfected cell lines producing recFSH have been established by transfection of CHO cells (CHO K1; ATCC CCL 61) with plasmids containing the two subunit genes encoding FSH, i.e. hCGα and FSHβ (11). The nucleotide sequences of the coding regions were identical to those described previously (14, 15). Transcription of the α gene is directed from the simian virus-40 promoter, whereas the β gene is transcribed from the human metallothionein-II_A promoter. Stable integration of the plasmid in the chromosomal DNA was verified by Southern blot analyses of total cellular DNA. A single cell clone producing FSH at a constant level was selected and used for large scale production via continuous perfusion.

Hormones and monoclonal antibodies (MCAs)

Highly purified (≥99%) (13) lyophilized recFSH (batch 63, 65 and ML-FSH-95) was supplied by Diosynth (Oss, The Netherlands), and hCG

(Pregnyl) was supplied by NV Organon (Oss, The Netherlands). Purified iodinated pituitary human FSH ($[^{125}I]$FSH; 3.3–7.4 megabecquerels (MBq)/μg) and [1β-^{3}H]androstenedione (1 TBq/mmol) were purchased from New England Nuclear-DuPont (Boston, MA). The International Standard (IS) of urinary human gonadotropins (code no. 70/45; 54 IU FSH and 46 IU LH per ampoule according to *in vivo* bioassays) and the IS of pituitary human FSH (code no. 83/575; 80 IU highly purified FSH/ampoule according to *in vivo* bioassay) were gifts from the National Institute of Biological Standards and Control (NIBSC, Hertfordshire, United Kingdom). Urinary FSH references were pure FSH (Metrodin, batches 88F02, 88I05, 89E16, 89J30, and 07325089, Serono, Rome, Italy), hMG 3/1 (batch Hu 332, Organon), and hMG 1/1 (Humegon, batches 08–2023–105, 890405–017, 881017–030, and 002025–105, Organon). The declared FSH/LH ratios of these three preparations according to *in vivo* bioassays were 60, 3, and 1, respectively. The FSH and hCG doses applied in *in vivo* experiments refer to their *in vivo* bioactivities as declared by the manufacturers (16, 17), which is in terms of IS 70/45 for recFSH, pure FSH, and hMG and in terms of the Third IS for hCG (code no. 75/537) for hCG. The protein content of FSH preparations was estimated from absorbance measurements at 280 nm of their solutions, assuming that $A_{1cm}^{1\%}$ 280 = 10.0 (18). MCAs (48A and 4B) raised against recFSH and urinary FSH, respectively, were developed by Organon. One MCA (INN-117) raised against pituitary FSH was a gift from Prof. G. Wick (Innsbruck, Austria).

Animals

Rats and mice were purchased from Harlan CPB (Zeist, The Netherlands) and housed at 21 °C (hypophysectomized animals at 25 °C), with intervals of 14 h of light and 10 h of darkness. The animals had free access to standard pelleted food (Hope Farms, Woerden, The Netherlands) and tap water.

Immunoassay for FSH

FSH immunoreactivity was measured in a sandwich enzyme immunoassay using a β-directed capturing MCA (4B) and an α-directed horseradish peroxidase-labeled detection MCA (116B). This assay, recognizing only intact dimers, is known to recognize all *in vitro* bioactive recFSH isoforms (13). The assay sensitivity using IS–70/45 was 0.4 IU/liter, and the intra- and interassay coefficients of variation were 7% and 8%, respectively. The cross-reactivities of the FSH immunoassay were less than 0.001% with hCG and less than 0.01% with hLH.

Receptor assay for FSH

This assay was based on the displacement of iodinated pituitary human FSH from calf testicular membrane preparations, by unlabeled FSH preparations.

The procedure of preparing partially purified membrane receptors was adapted from that of Abou-Issa and Reichert (19). In brief, fresh bovine testes from calves (4–5 months of age) were collected on ice and stored at −80 °C. The decapsulated testes were homogenized in ice-cold 0.25 M sucrose in 10 mM Tris–HCl, pH 7.4, containing 5 mM $MgCl_2$ (3 ml/g tissue) with a Polytron homogenizer (Brinkmann, Westbury, NY) at maximum speed for 60 sec. The homogenate was filtered through two layers of mesh grid and centrifuged (10 min; $200 \times g$; 4 °C). The supernatant was further centrifuged at $15,000 \times g$ (30 min; 4 °C). The pellet was resuspended in 10 mM Tris–HCl, pH 7.4, containing 5 mM $MgCl_2$ (1 ml/g starting tissue). Protein content was determined by the method of Bradford (20), using BSA (Sigma, St. Louis, MO) as a standard. Testicular membrane fractions (50 µg protein/200 µl assay buffer; 10 mM Tris–HCl, pH 7.4, supplemented with 5 mM $MgCl_2$ and 1 g/liter BSA) were incubated with [^{125}I]FSH (50,000 cpm/200 µl) and FSH sample (100 µl). After 24 h of incubation at room temperature, 500 µl ice-cold assay buffer were added, and bound and free hormone were separated by centrifugation ($15,000 \times g$; 5 min). Radioactivity in the pellet was measured using a LKB γ-counter (Rockville, MD). Data were expressed as the percentage bound divided by the total added counts.

In vitro bioassays for FSH and LH

In vitro FSH and LH bioassays were based on induction of aromatase activity in immature rat Sertoli cells (21) and induction of testosterone production in mouse Leydig cells (22), respectively. The procedures of these assays were described previously (23).

In brief, Sertoli cells were collected from 10-day-old Wistar rats and cultured in 24-well plates (Costar, Cambridge, MA) for 3 days at 37 °C in a humidified atmosphere of 5% CO_2–95% air. Culture medium consisted of a 1:1 (vol/vol) mixture of Ham's F-12 and Dulbecco's Modified Eagle's Medium supplemented with 5 µg/ml bovine insulin (Diosynth) and 5 mg/ml human transferrin (Sigma). After an initial culture period, each well was washed and incubated under the same conditions for 18 h with 1 ml of the above-described culture medium containing 0.2 mM 3-isobutyl-1-methylxanthine (Aldrich-Europe, Beerse, Belgium), 1 g/liter BSA, and FSH test sample. For the testing of MCAs, FSH and MCAs were preincubated for 1 h at room temperature.

The FSH dose chosen gave a just maximal response in the absence of MCAs.

Aromatase activity was assessed by measuring the release of ^3H_2O from [1β-^{3}H]androstenedione. Therefore, the culture plates were incubated for 4 h (37 °C) with Dulbecco's PBS (Gibco Europe, Breda, The Netherlands) containing 5.6 mM glucose and labeled androstenedione (37 kBq/ml/well; 0.22 µM). Supernatants were extracted with 5 ml chloroform, and the aqueous phase was treated with a suspension of 50 g/liter Norit-A (Sigma) and 5 g/liter Dextran T-70 (Pharmacia, Uppsala, Sweden) in distilled water. The radioactivity of the supernatant fraction was measured by a liquid scintillation counter (Packard, Zurich, Switzerland).

Leydig cells were isolated from the testes of mature Swiss mice (9–13 weeks old). The cells were obtained by sucking each decapsulated testis five times through a glass tube and filtering the suspension through a 30-µm nylon mesh. The cells were suspended in medium 199 supplemented with 4.2 mM $NaHCO_3$, 20 ml/liter fetal calf serum (Gibco-Europe), and 1 g/liter BSA, and 100 µl cell suspension were added to each well of a microtiter plate (Greiner, Nurtingen, Germany) along with a 50 µl test sample. Plates were incubated for 4 h at 37 °C in a humidified atmosphere of 5% CO_2–95% air and subsequently stored at −20 °C until testosterone determination by RIA.

In vivo experiments

Four days after hypophysectomy, immature female Wistar rats (45–50 g; six or seven animals per treatment group) were treated for 4 days by twice daily sc injections of recFSH only (total dose, 5, 10, 20, or 40 IU) or recFSH (total dose, 40 IU) supplemented with various doses of hCG (total doses, 0, 0.1, 1, and 10 IU) or with hCG only (total dose, 1 or 10 IU). In a comparable way, animals were treated with urinary FSH preparations, *viz.* pure FSH, hMG 3/1, or hMG 1/1. Control animals were injected with vehicle solution only, consisting of 43.7 mM NaH_2PO_4, 109.7 mM Na_2HPO_4, 1 g/liter methylhydroxybenzoate, and 1 g/liter gelatin. Animals were killed 18 h after the last injection. After diethyl ether anesthesia, the rats were exsanguinated, and their ovaries were dissected out, weighed, and frozen at −80 °C until determinations of aromatase activity. For that purpose, ovaries were thawed, minced by scissors, and homogenized with a Potter-Elvejhem homogenizer in ice-cold 0.1 M potassium phosphate buffer supplemented with 5 mM EDTA. The final tissue concentration was 1 mg/ml. After centrifugation at 300×g for 10 min at 0 °C, 5 µl of an ethanolic solution of [1β-^{3}H]androstenedione (37 kBq/incubate; 74 nM) were added to 0.9 ml supernatant, and the incubation was started by adding 0.1 ml of a NADPH-generating system. The final concentrations in the incubate were 2.5 mM NADP, 5 mM glucose-6-phosphate, and 0.525 U/ml glucose-6-phosphate dehydrogenase. The incubation was performed at 37 °C for 15 min and terminated by adding 5 ml chloroform and thoroughly mixing. The ^3H_2O content in the aqueous phase was assessed as described above.

For histological examination, ovaries were fixed in formal sublimate, dehydrated, and embedded in paraffin. Serial sections (10 μm) were stained with hemalum and eosin.

Steroid assessments

Testosterone was established in a direct RIA kit (Farmos Diagnostica, Oulunsal, Finland), using a calibration curve of standard testosterone doses in Leydig cell culture medium. Estradiol in rat plasma samples was assayed in an 17β-estradiol kit (ICN Biomedicals, Inc., Carson, CA) after solid phase extraction using octadecyl columns (Baker, Deventer, The Netherlands). Androstenedione in supernatants of rat ovarian homogenates was determined using a direct androstenedione kit (Diagnostic Systems Laboratories, Inc., Webster, TX).

Statistical analysis

Potencies relative to the standard were calculated after testing for linearity and parallelism of the dose–response curves, as described by Finney (24).

Statistical analysis of responses in hypophysectomized rats was performed according to a complete randomized design, and significance was defined as $P < 0.05$. Responses of ovarian weight and aromatase activity were analyzed by one-way variance analysis after log transformation of the original data. Median estradiol levels were tested in the Wilcoxon sum of ranks test.

RESULTS

Specific FSH activity

Specific FSH activities (international units per mg protein) of recFSH, pituitary FSH (IS 83/575), urinary pure FSH (Metrodin), and hMG 1/1 (Humegon) according to immunoassay and *in vivo* bioassay were calculated after estimation of their protein contents from absorbance measurements at 280 nm. The calculated activities, expressed in terms of IS 70/45, are presented in Table 1. The specific *in vivo* bio- and immunoactivities of recFSH were considerably higher than those of pure FSH (Metrodin) and hMG 1/1 (Humegon), but the *in vivo* bio/immuno ratios of these preparations were not significantly different. When compared to the highly purified pituitary standard IS 83/575, recFSH and IS 83/575 had comparable high specific *in vivo* bioactivities, but the specific immunoreactivity of IS 83/575 was about 2 times lower, resulting in a significantly increased *in vivo*/immuno ratio.

In vitro receptor binding and bioactivity

The receptor affinity and *in vitro* bioactivity of recFSH were examined in receptor displacement studies using calf testicular membranes and in bioassay studies using immature rat Sertoli cells. In these experiments recFSH provided dose–response curves parallel to those of pituitary and urinary FSH references.

When equal amounts of immunoreactive FSH were tested, recFSH, urinary pure FSH (Metrodin), hMG 1/1 (Humegon), and pituitary FSH (IS 83/575) inhibited the receptor binding of pituitary [^{125}I]FSH in a dose-dependent manner and in the same dose range.

RecFSH, urinary FSH (IS 70/45), and pituitary FSH (IS 83/575) increased the aromatase activity in rat Sertoli cells in a dose-dependent manner (Figure 1, *lower panel*). Like receptor-binding potencies, *in vitro* bioactivities of recFSH and natural FSH references were comparable. Also, recFSH and natural FSH induced comparable maximal responses in all experiments.

In vitro neutralization of bioactivity

The capacity of anti-FSH antibodies to inhibit the *in vitro* bioactivity of recFSH was investigated by means of three MCAs raised against urinary FSH (MCA 4β; β-specific), pituitary FSH (MCA INN-117; αβ-specific), or recFSH (MCA 48A; α-specific). In the Sertoli cell bioassay, each MCA inhibited the aromatase activity induced by recFSH. Moreover, the amounts of MCA needed to neutralize the *in vitro* bioactivity of pure FSH, pituitary FSH (IS 83/575) and recFSH were comparable. To obtain 50% inhibition of responses induced by immunoreactive FSH doses of 6.4 IU recFSH, 7.9 IU pure FSH, or 7.8 IU pituitary FSH (IS 83/575), 4 nM MCA 4B, 0.1 nM MCA INN-117, and 0.08 nM MCA 48A in total were required. As a typical example, the results of one neutralization experiment with MCA 48A are shown in Figure 2.

Table 1 Specific FSH activity (international units per mg protein; mean with 95% confidence limits) of recFSH and natural FSH references according to *in vivo* bioassay and immunoassay in terms of the urinary IS 70/45

Preparation	n	In vivo bioactivity	Immunoreactivity	In vivo/immuno ratio
RecFSH	3	14,000 (12,100–15,900)	12,100 (11,100–14,900)	1.2 (0.8–1.4)
IS 83/575	1	14,100 (12,500–15,800)	5,600 (5,400–5,900)	2.5 (2.1–2.9)
Pure FSH	2	221[a] (177–276)	180 (168–192)	1.2 (0.9–1.6)
hMG 1/1	3	65[a] (52–81)	42 (40–43)	1.5 (1.2–2.0)
IS 70/45	1	54[b]		

n represents the number of batches tested.
[a] Assuming 75 (60–94) IU *in vivo* bioactive FSH/ampoule, as stated by the manufacturers.
[b] Taken from Storring *et al.* (25).

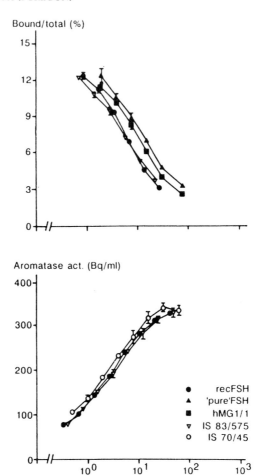

Figure 1 Dose-dependent displacement of labeled human pituitary [^{125}I]FSH binding to calf testicular membranes (*upper panel*) and stimulation of aromatase activity in immature rat Sertoli cells (*lower panel*) by recFSH produced by CHO cells and natural FSH references. Responses represent the mean of triplicates ± SD

Intrinsic LH activity

To establish whether recFSH is capable of inducing LH-specific biological responses, an *in vitro* mouse Leydig cell testosterone bioassay was applied. Figure 3 shows the induction of testosterone synthesis by urinary IS 70/45, urinary pure FSH, and recFSH. While 0.2–6 IU pure FSH induced dose responses parallel to those of IS 70/45, 16–64 IU recFSH were needed to increase testosterone production. The calculated *in vitro* LH activity in terms of IS 70/45 per IU *in vivo* bioactive FSH was

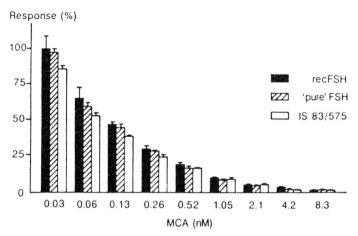

Figure 2 Inhibition of FSH-induced aromatase activity in immature rat Sertoli cells. Increasing doses of MCA 48A were preincubated for 1 h at room temperature with one FSH dose, causing nearly maximal aromatase activity in the absence of MCA. Responses represent the mean of triplicates ± SD

2.4 (2.2–2.7) mIU LH/IU FSH for pure FSH (Metrodin batch 88F02) and less than 0.025 mIU LH/IU FSH for recFSH.

In vivo bioactivities

The *in vivo* efficacy of recFSH was established by treating immature hypophysectomized female rats for 4 days with either recFSH only or recFSH supplemented with 1 IU hCG. The FSH and hCG dosages applied in these animal experiments represent their *in vivo* bioactivities.

Total dosages of 5, 10, 20, and 40 IU recFSH increased ovarian weight and ovarian aromatase activity in a dose-dependent manner (Figure 4). Both responses were significantly ($P < 0.05$) increased by a total dose of 5 IU recFSH, while at least 20 IU were needed to reach maximal responses. Gross histological examination of ovaries after treatment with 10 IU recFSH revealed the presence of large antral follicles, while in vehicle-injected animals, only primordial and primary follicles were observed. When the various recFSH dosages were supplemented with 1 IU hCG, both ovarian weight and aromatase activity were further augmented ($P < 0.05$), especially at recFSH dosages that produced submaximal responses. Treatment with 1 IU hCG alone did not affect these parameters.

In the absence of hCG, as much as 40 IU recFSH was unable to increase plasma estradiol levels, while recFSH supplemented with 1 IU hCG largely increased median plasma estradiol levels in a FSH dose-

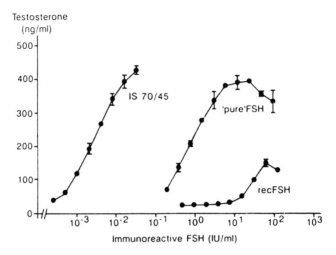

Figure 3 Stimulation of testosterone production in mouse Leydig cells by increasing doses of recFSH and urinary FSH preparations. Responses represent the mean of quadruplicates ± SD

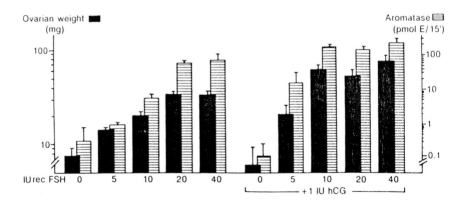

Figure 4 Ovarian weight and ovarian aromatase activity in immature hypophysectomized rats ($n = 6$–7) after treatment with increasing doses of recFSH alone or in combination with 1 IU hCG. Responses represent the geometric mean ± SEM

Table 2 Median plasma 17β-estradiol levels in immature hypophysectomized rats after FSH treatment

Treatment	Total dose (IU) FSH	LH/hCG	Estradiol (pg/ml)
RecFSH only	0		8.9
	5		10.4
	10		9.6
	20		10.0
	40		10.8
RecFSH + hCG	0	1	3.6
	5	1	93.8
	10	1	95.7
	20	1	200
	40	1	454
RecFSH + hCG	40	0	10.9
	40	0.1	34.3
	40	1	674
	40	10	1090
	0	10	5.2
Pure FSH	40	≤0.7	9.0
hMG 3/1	40	13	527
hMG 1/1	40	40	1440

Four days after hypophysectomy, rats (six or seven animals per treatment group) were treated for 4 days by twice daily sc injections of recFSH only and recFSH supplemented with hCG, urinary pure FSH, hMG 3/1, and hMG 1/1.

dependent manner (Table 2). Animals treated with 1 IU hCG only had unchanged basal estradiol levels.

To estimate how much LH activity would be needed to increase plasma estradiol levels in the above-described experimental model, animals were treated with recFSH in addition to 0, 0.1, 1, or 10 IU hCG, and pure FSH, hMG 3/1, and hMG 1/1 were used as references. All animals received 40 IU *in vivo* bioactive FSH, since this dose of recFSH was known to induce maximal aromatase activity. Effects of endogenous androstenedione levels in rat ovaries on the assessment of aromatase were negligible, even after treatment with the highest dose hCG or hMG 1/1, since these levels were less than 5% of the total amount of substrate used.

Increases in ovarian weight and aromatase activity induced by recFSH only and urinary pure FSH were not significantly different

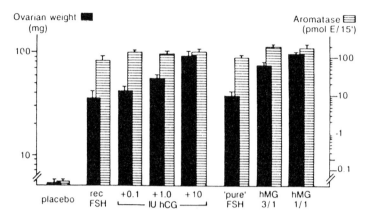

Figure 5 Ovarian weight and aromatase activity in immature hypophysectomized rats ($n = 6$–7) after treatment with a total of 40 IU FSH or recFSH alone or in combination with hCG (0.1, 1, or 10 IU), urinary pure FSH (batch 89E16), hMG 3/1, and hMG 1/1. Responses represent the geometric mean ± SEM

(Figure 5). When recFSH was supplemented with 1 and 10 IU hCG, increases in ovarian weight and aromatase were further augmented ($P < 0.05$) and comparable to those induced by hMG 3/1 and hMG 1/1, respectively. In comparison to controls, animals treated with 10 IU hCG only had slightly increased ($P < 0.05$) ovarian weights and aromatase activity (data not shown).

Like recFSH, urinary pure FSH was unable to increase circulating estradiol levels (Table 2). However, when recFSH was supplemented with hCG, recFSH largely increased circulating estradiol levels in a hCG dose-dependent manner. As little as 0.1 IU hCG produced a 3-fold increase in median estradiol levels, while these levels remained unchanged after treatment with 10 IU hCG alone. The estradiol levels induced by recFSH supplemented with 1 and 10 IU hCG compared well with those induced by hMG 3/1 and hMG 1/1, respectively.

DISCUSSION

In the present study the *in vitro* and *in vivo* biological properties of recFSH produced by CHO cells were compared to those of natural FSH preparations. In this study recFSH was the only preparation tested with a biochemical purity of at least 99% (13); all natural FSH preparations were contaminated with small or large amounts of other proteins from pituitary or urinary origin. For this reason, a comparison of preparations based on the amount of FSH protein was not feasible; dose uniformity of the various FSH preparations was obtained by their calibration in terms of IS 70/45 in immunoassay and *in vivo* bioassay for the purpose of comparative *in vitro* and *in vivo* experiments, respectively.

The high specific activities (>10,100 IU/mg protein) or recFSH, determined by immunoassay and *in vivo* bioassay, support the high purity of the preparation tested. In the present study all estimations of protein content were based on the absorbance of FSH solutions at 280 nm. When applying protein assays based on different principles of protein recognition and/or using various protein standards, the specific activity of recFSH ranged between 10.000–40.000 IU/mg protein (data not shown).

Measurement of specific *in vivo* bioactivity and immunoreactivity revealed that the *in vivo*/immuno ratios of recFSH and urinary FSH were not different, indicating that the isohormone profiles of these two types of preparations are very similar (13). The *in vivo*/immuno ratio of the highly purified IS 83/575 appeared to be about 2 times higher than those of the other tested FSH preparations. This finding is in good agreement with the previous reported discrepancy of the declared *in vivo* bioactivity (80 IU/ampoule) and the much lower actual immunoreactivity of this IS (18). In general, the acidic FSH isoforms contribute far more to the *in vivo* bioactivity than to the *in vitro* bioactivity or immunoreactivity (26). Therefore, these data suggest that IS 83/575 contains relatively more acidic isoforms than the other tested FSH preparations. Since one would expect pituitary FSH to be less acidic than urinary FSH, it might well be that this IS 83/575 has lost considerable amounts of basic isoforms during purification.

The data of receptor displacement assays and *in vitro* bioassays revealed that recFSH and the tested natural FSH references have similar *in vitro* activities, meaning that the immuno/*in vitro* ratios of these preparations are similar. Previous reports on *in vitro* bioactive recFSH produced by CHO cells were based on induction of aromatase activity in rat granulosa cells (27, 28). In the present study the functional effect of recFSH was established by means of an *in vitro* Sertoli cell aromatase bioassay. Like the granulosa cell bioassay, this assay has demonstrated its suitability for FSH quantification of gonadotropin preparations and serum samples (23, 29–31).

The *in vitro* induction of aromatase activity could be inhibited by preincubation of recFSH or urinary or pituitary FSH with MCAs raised against either of these FSH preparations. The almost identical neutralization profiles of recombinant and natural FSH in various experiments using MCAs directed against three different FSH epitopes supports the structural and functional similarity of both types of molecules.

One of the obvious advantages of recFSH is that it does not contain other hormones, such as LH. By means of the Leydig cell bioassay, it was demonstrated that the intrinsic LH bioactivity of recFSH is negligible; the amounts of recFSH needed to increase *in vitro* testosterone production were extremely high and clearly supraphysiological.

The first report (4) supporting the two-cell two-gonadotropin theory was made about 50 yr ago. It demonstrated that highly purified FSH could increase ovarian growth and follicular development in immature hypophysectomized rats without stimulating the release of estrogen, since uterine weights remained unchanged. These findings were confirmed by some investigators (5, 6), while others (32) reported increases in both ovarian and uterine weights. Since increases in uterine weight are thought to reflect both FSH and LH activities and may also be due to nonspecific factors (17), previous studies using natural FSH were not conclusive.

The present study provides more definite evidence in favor of the two-cell theory, confirming that FSH alone can stimulate follicular growth and that LH activity is required to increase estradiol secretion up to measurable plasma levels. Like recFSH, urinary pure FSH was unable to increase circulating estradiol, while a combination of recFSH and 0.1 IU hCG (<2.5 mIU hCG/IU FSH) provided a 3-fold increase in median plasma estradiol levels. Obviously, the remaining LH activity in pure FSH (2–3 mIU LH/IU FSH) was insufficient to increase circulating estradiol, which could be due to the much shorter elimination half-life of LH than of hCG (33). Our findings in hypophysectomized rats seem to be in disagreement with those in higher species demonstrating that gonadotropin-suppressed subjects may have normal rising estradiol levels in response to urinary pure FSH (7). However, up to now, neither GnRH agonists nor antagonists have been shown to establish complete pituitary suppression (34), and remaining endogenous LH secretion as well as ovarian androgens might be sufficient to cause increases in estradiol.

The ability of recFSH to induce follicular growth in hypophysectomized rats has recently also been demonstrated by Galway *et al.* (35). Moreover, their experiments indicate that recFSH alone is able to induce ovulation. This suggests that FSH-induced synthesis of ovarian estradiol and/or growth factors is sufficient for complete follicle maturation, although the quality of oocytes and their progeny remains to be investigated. Our study also demonstrated that recFSH supplemented with hCG causes much higher increases in ovarian weight and aromatase activity than treatment with recFSH only when using recFSH doses that provided submaximal responses. The effect of LH activity on ovarian aromatase is known to be mediated via testosterone and 5α-reduced androgens, causing amplification of cAMP-mediated FSH responses (36). Thus, while LH might not play a crucial role in follicular maturation, it remains obvious that LH supports and augments the regulatory function of FSH during folliculogenesis.

In summary, the present study shows by means of various *in vitro* and *in vivo* models that the biological properties of recFSH produced by CHO cells are very similar, if not identical, to those of natural FSH preparations.

ACKNOWLEDGEMENTS

We gratefully acknowledge the technical assistance of Mr. C. Strijbos, his co-workers, Ms. I. Grijsbach, Ms. L. Hellings, Mr. F. Wijnands, and Mr. E. Lammers. We are indebted to Dr. P. Schot for attending the histotechnical work, and to Mr. F. Verbon for statistical analysis of the data. We also wish to thank Prof. G. Wick (Innsbruck) for his generous gift of MCA INN-117.

REFERENCES

1. Sharp RM 1990 Intratesticular control of steroidogenesis. Clin Endocrinol (Oxf) 33:787–807
2. Hsueh AJW, Adashi EY, Jones PBC, Welsh TH 1984 Hormonal regulation of the differentiation of cultured ovarian granulosa cells. Endocr Rev 5:76–127
3. Dorrington JH, Armstrong DT 1979 Effects of FSH on gonadal functions. Recent Prog Horm Res 35:301–342
4. Fevold HL 1941 Synergism of follicle stimulating and luteinizing hormone in producing estrogen secretion. Endocrinology 28:33–36
5. Greep RO, VanDyke HB, Chow BF 1942 Gonadotropins of the swine pituitary. I. Various biological effects of purified thylakentrin (FSH) and pure metakentrin (ICSH). Endocrinology 30:635–649
6. Lohstroh AJ, Johnson RE 1966 Amounts of interstitial cell-stimulating hormone and follicle-stimulating hormone required for follicular development uterine growth and ovulation in the hypophysectomized rat. Endocrinology 79:991–996
7. Hodgen GD 1989 Biological basis of follicle growth. Hum Reprod 4:37–46
8. Kenigsberg D, Littman BA, Williams RF, Hodgen GD 1984 Medical hypophysectomy. II. Variability of ovarian responses to gonadotropin therapy. Fertil Steril 42:116–126
9. Edelstein MC, Brzyski RG, Jones GS, Simonetti S, Muasher SJ 1990 Equivalence of human menopausal gonadotropin and follicle-stimulating hormone stimulation after gonadotropin-releasing hormone against suppression. Fertil Steril 53:103–106

10. Couzinet B, Lestrat N, Brailly S, Forest M, Schaison G 1988 Stimulation of ovarian follicular maturation with pure follicle-stimulating hormone in women with gonadotropin deficiency. J Clin Endocrinol Metab 66:552–556
11. Van Wezenbeek P, Draaier J, Van Meel F, Olijve W 1990 Recombinant follicle stimulating hormone. I. Construction, selection and characterization of a cell line. In: Crommelin DJA, Schellekens H (eds) From Clone to Clinic, Developments in Biotherapy. Kluwer, Dordrecht, vol 1:245–251
12. Hård K, Mekking A, Damm JBL, Kamerling JP, de Boer W, Wijnands RA, Vliegenthart JFG 1990 Isolation and structure determination of the intact sialylated N-linked carbohydrate chains of recombinant human follitropin (hFSH) expressed in Chinese hamster ovary cells. Eur J Biochem 193:263–271
13. De Boer W, Mannaerts B 1990 Recombinant follicle stimulating hormone. II. Biochemical and biological characteristics. In: Crommelin DJA, Schellekens H (eds) From Clone to Clinic, Developments in Biotherapy. Kluwer, Dordrecht, vol 1:253–259
14. Fiddes JC, Goodman HW 1981 The genes encoding the common alpha subunit of the four human glycoprotein hormones. J Mol Appl Genet 1:3–18
15. Jameson JL, Becker CB, Lindell CM, Habener JF 1988 Human follicle stimulating hormone β-subunit gene encodes multiple messenger ribonucleic acids. Mol Endocrinol 2:806–815
16. Steelman SL, Pohley FM 1953 Assay of the follicle stimulating hormone based on the augmentation with human chorionic gonadotropin. Endocrinology 53:604–616
17. Van Hell H, Matthijsen R, Overbeek GA 1964 Effects of human menopausal gonadotrophin preparations in different bioassay methods. Acta Endocrinol (Copenh) 47:409–418
18. Storring PL, Gaines Das RE 1989 The international standard for pituitary FSH: collaborative study of the standard and of four other purified human FSH preparations of differing molecular composition by bioassays, receptor assays and different immunoassay systems. J Endocrinol 123:275–293
19. Abou-Issa H, Reichert LE 1977 Solubilization and some characteristics of the follitropin receptor from calf testis. J Biol Chem 252:4166–4174
20. Bradford M 1976 A rapid and sensitive method for the quantitation of microgram quantities of protein utilizing the principle of protein-dye binding. Anal Biochem 72:248–254
21. Van Damme MP, Robertson DM, Marana R, Ritzen EM, Diczfalusy E 1979 A sensitive and specific *in vitro* bioassay method for the measurement of follicle-stimulating hormone activity. Acta Endocrinol (Copenh) 91:224–237
22. Van Damme MP, Robertson DM, Diczfalusy E 1974 An improved *in vitro* bioassay for measuring luteinizing hormone (LH) activity using mouse Leydig cell preparations. Acta Endocrinol (Copenh) 77:655–671
23. Mannaerts BMJL, Kloosterboer HJ, Schuurs AHWM 1987 Applications of *in vitro* bioassays for gonadotrophins. In: Rolland R, Heineman MJ, Naaktgeboren N, Schoemaker J, Vemer H, Willemsen WNP (eds) Neuro-

Endocrinology of Reproduction. Exerpt Med Int Congr Ser 751, Elsevier, Amsterdam, pp 49–58
24. Finney DJ 1978 Statistical Method in Biological Assay, ed 3. Griffin, London
25. Storring PL, Dixon H, Bangham DR 1976 The first international standard for human urinary FSH and for human urinary LH (ICSH), for bioassay. Acta Endocrinol (Copenh) 83:700–710
26. Ulloa-Aquirre A, Espinoza R, Damian-Matsumura P, Chappel SC 1988 Immunological and biological potencies of different molecular species of gonadotrophins. Hum Reprod 3:491–501
27. Keene JL, Matzuk MM, Otani T, Fauser BCJM, Galway AB, Hsueh AJW, Biome I 1989 Expression of biologically active human follitropin in Chinese hamster ovary cells. J Biol Chem 246:4769–4775
28. Galway AB, Hsueh AJW, Keene JL, Yamoto M, Fauser BCJM, Boime I 1990 *In vitro* and *in vivo* bioactivity of recombinant human follicle-stimulating hormone and partially deglycosylated variants secreted by transfected eukaryotic cell lines. Endocrinology 127:93–100
29. Padmanabhan V, Chappel SC, Beitins IZ 1987 An improved *in vitro* bioassay for follicle-stimulating hormone suitable for measurement of FSH in unextracted serum. Endocrinology 121:1089–1098
30. Padmanabhan V, Lang L, Sonstein J, Klech RP, Beitins IZ 1988 Modulation of serum follicle-stimulating hormone bioactivity and isoform distribution by estrogenic steroids in normal women and in gonadal dysgenesis. J Clin Endocrinol Metab 67:465–473
31. Jockenhövel F, Khan SA, Nieschlag E 1989 Diagnostic value of bioactive FSH in male infertility. Acta Endocrinol (Copenh) 121:802–810
32. Papkoff H 1965 Some biological properties of a potent follicle stimulating hormone preparation. Acta Endocrinol (Copenh) 48:439–445
33. Yen SSC, Llerena LA, Little B, Pearson OH 1968 Disappearance rates of endogenous luteinizing hormone and chorionic gonadotropin in man. J Clin Endocrinol Metab 30:325–329
34. Loumaye E 1990 The control of endogenous secretion of LH by gonadotrophin-releasing hormone agonists during ovarian hyper-stimulation for *in-vitro* fertilization and embryo transfer. Hum Reprod 5:357–376
35. Galway AB, Lapolt PS, Tsafriri A, Dargan CM, Boime I, Hsueh AJW 1990 Recombinant follicle-stimulating hormone induces ovulation and tissue plasminogen activator expression in hypophysectomized rats. Endocrinology 127:3023–3028
36. Hillier SG 1990 Ovarian manipulation with pure gonadotrophins. J Endocrinol 127:1–4

Received March 8, 1991

Correspondence: Bernadette Mannaerts, Medical R&D Unit, NV Organon, PO Box 20, 5340 BH Oss, The Netherlands

2

Effects of recombinant human follicle stimulating hormone on cultured human granulosa cells: comparison with urinary gonadotrophins and actions in preovulatory follicles

H.D. Mason*, B.M.J.L. Mannaerts[†], R. de Leeuw[†], D.S. Willis* and S. Franks*

*Department of Obstetrics and Gynaecology, Imperial College of Science Technology and Medicine, St Mary's Hospital Medical School, London W2 1PG, UK and [†]Scientific Development Group, NV Organon, 5340 BH Oss, The Netherlands

ABSTRACT

The effects of recombinant human follicle stimulating hormone (rFSH; Org 32489) have been examined in human granulosa cells from ovaries obtained from women with spontaneous menses. In the first series of experiments the actions of rFSH on production of oestradiol and progesterone were compared with those of urinary-derived gonadotrophins. Recombinant FSH induced dose-dependent increases in production of both oestradiol and progesterone which were similar to the effects of 'pure' FSH (Metrodin®) and the International Standard IS 71/223. In further studies, the actions of rFSH on oestradiol production by individual preovulatory follicles were investigated; rFSH increased oestradiol accumulation from cells obtained from follicles before the luteinizing hormone (LH) surge. In contrast, rFSH inhibited oestradiol production by granulosa cells derived from a follicle after the onset of the LH surge, whereas the gonadotrophic action of growth hormone was maintained. Following preliminary reports of the in-vivo effects of rFSH in women, these findings provide further validation of the efficacy of rFSH in the human ovary. The results of studies of the preovulatory follicle illustrate the experimental importance of the availability of recombinant preparations of pure gonadotrophins, produced by recombinant technology, in the understanding of human ovarian function.

INTRODUCTION

The relative contributions of follicle stimulating hormone (FSH) and luteinizing hormone (LH) to folliculogenesis have been a subject of interest and discussion for many years. In recent years, in-vitro experiments with isolated granulosa and theca cells have provided further insight into the diverse molecular mechanisms by which FSH and LH regulate ovarian function (Hsueh *et al.*, 1984; Gore-Langton and Armstrong, 1988; Hillier, 1991). Nevertheless, interpretation of the results of such studies has been complicated by the lack of purity of the preparations of LH and FSH tested. More recently, pure FSH has become available through the application of recombinant DNA technology. Using recombinant human FSH (rFSH, Org 32489), experiments in animals have demonstrated that receptor-binding affinity, in-vitro and in-vivo bioactivities were comparable to those of natural FSH preparations (Mannaerts *et al.*, 1991). Receptor studies, however, suggest that the properties of the human gonadotrophin receptors may differ from those of experimental animals (Alpaugh *et al.*, 1990; Jia *et al.*, 1991; Tilly *et al.*, 1992), thus emphasizing the importance of investigating the specific interaction of rFSH with its homologous receptor.

In the current study, rFSH-mediated effects in human granulosa cells of small antral follicles were examined and compared with the actions of FSH isolated from natural sources. Subsequent experiments were designed to examine the specific action of FSH on granulosa cells from preovulatory follicles. The final stages of maturation of the dominant follicle are characterized by acquisition of functional LH receptors, and production of oestradiol becomes dependent not only on FSH but also on LH (Yong *et al.*, 1992). It remains unclear, however, whether the preovulatory follicle remains responsive to FSH after the onset of the LH surge. The availability of a pure (LH-free) FSH preparation affords the opportunity to investigate the effects of FSH alone in follicles at this stage of development.

Table 1 Details of patients included in the study. Patient 2 had had a previous total abdominal hysterectomy (TAH)

Patient	Figure	Age (years)	Cycle history	No. of follicles pooled (size range, mm)
1	1	46	regular	3 (7–15)
2	2	39	TAH (previously regular)	14 (5–10)
3	3, 5(left)	42	oligomenorrhoea	1 (20)
4	4, 5(right)	42	oligomenorrhoea	1 (20)

MATERIALS AND METHODS

Human granulosa cell cultures

Ovaries were obtained from four patients with spontaneous menstrual cycles who were undergoing surgery for non-ovarian gynaecological disease (Table 1). Follicles were dissected intact from the surrounding stroma, and granulosa cells scraped from the theca interna. Cells were then washed, subjected to gentle mechanical dispersion and plated at a density of ~50 000 viable cells per well, as previously described (Mason et al., 1990a). Cells from smaller follicles were pooled but those from preovulatory follicles provided sufficient granulosa cells to study the steroid production in individual follicles (Table 1). Incubations were performed for 48 h in serum-free Medium 199 (Gibco BRL, Paisley, UK) in the presence of 10^{-7} M testosterone with or without FSH. Cells from two large follicles were also incubated with testosterone and a range of doses of growth hormone with or without the addition of FSH.

Hormones

The following gonadotrophins were used in the various experiments. Pure (99.9%) lyophilised rFSH (Org 32489, batch 65) with a specific in-vivo bioactivity of 13 100 (range 12 100–14 300) IU/mg protein, was supplied by NV Organon (Oss, The Netherlands). Purified human pituitary FSH (code CPDSM1, <16 IU LH/mg) was kindly provided by Dr S. Lynch (Department of Endocrinology, Birmingham and Midland Hospital for Women, Birmingham, UK); and purified urinary FSH (urofollitrophin, Metrodin®, batch 91B21, 75 IU and <1 IU/LH/ampoule) was purchased from Serono (Rome, Italy). The first International Standard (IS) of urinary gonadotrophins (71/223) and the third

IS of human chorionic gonadotrophin (HCG, IS 75/537) were a gift from the National Institute of Biological Standards and Control (NIBSC, Hertfordshire, UK). CG, 75/537, was used in comparative studies to correct for the varying amounts of remaining LH activities in the test preparations. In these experiments, recombinant human insulin-like growth factor-I (IGF-I, Bissendorf, Hanover, Germany) was also added to augment oestradiol responsiveness to FSH (Erickson et al., 1989; Mason et al., 1993). Recombinant human growth hormone (Norditropin, Novo-Nordisk, Gentofte, Denmark; Mason et al., 1990b) was used in the studies on granulosa cells from preovulatory follicles.

Oestradiol and progesterone were measured in collected conditioned medium by radioimmunoassay (Mason et al., 1990a). Individual means were compared using Student's t-test.

RESULTS

Comparison of rFSH with urinary FSH preparations

Recombinant FSH produced a dose-related increase in oestradiol accumulation by granulosa cells from follicles of 7–15 mm (Figure 1). As shown in the left-hand panel of Figure 1, rFSH in the absence of testosterone consistently failed to stimulate oestradiol production in these experiments. Supplementation of the culture medium with HCG and

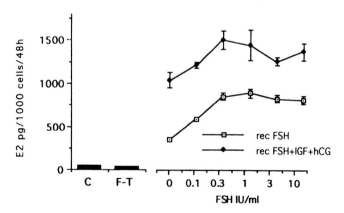

Figure 1 Oestradiol response to a range of doses of recombinant follicle stimulating hormone (rFSH) with or without the addition of insulin-like growth factor-I (IGF-I) (50 ng/ml) and human chorionic gonadotrophin (HCG) (30 ng/ml). C = incubation in medium alone, F–T = incubation with 1 IU/ml rFSH in the absence of testosterone. Values throughout the figures represent the mean ± SE of quadruplicate experiments

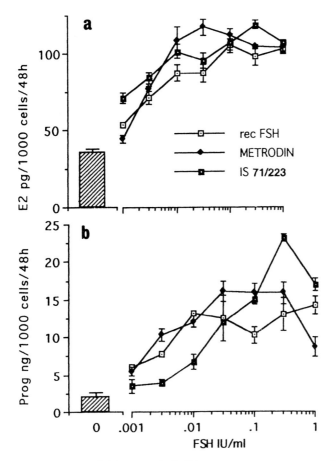

Figure 2 Comparison of (a) oestradiol, (b) progesterone response, by granulosa cells incubated with testosterone, insulin-like factor-I (IGF-I) and human chorionic gonadotrophin (HCG) with or without a range of doses of three follicle stimulating hormone (FSH) preparations. There were no significant differences between the preparations in oestradiol or progesterone production

IGF-I in the presence of testosterone resulted in an augmentation of estradiol secretion, although it did not improve the sensitivity of the assay system. All subsequent experiments comparing FSH preparations were performed with the addition of HCG and IGF-I (Figures 2 and 3). In the first of the comparative studies, the effects of rFSH on oestradiol production were observed to be similar to those of metrodin and IS 71/223 over the concentration range 0.03–100 IU/ml (data not shown). The maximum oestradiol response, representing an almost two-fold increase over baseline, was obtained at concentrations between 0.03 and 0.3 IU/ml. Therefore, in subsequent experiments, a

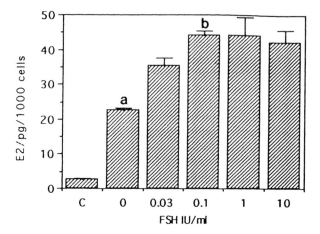

Figure 3 Stimulation of oestradiol production by recombinant follicle stimulating hormone (rFSH) in granulosa cells from a preovulatory follicle prior to the luteinizing hormone (LH) surge (a versus b, $P = 0.01$). C = medium alone

lower range of concentrations was studied. All three gonadotrophin preparations stimulated a dose-dependent increase in oestradiol concentrations in the dose range 0.001–0.03 IU/ml (Figure 2a). The three FSH preparations gave rise to comparable ED_{50} values: 2.9, 2.9 and 2.0 IU/l for rFSH, metrodin and IS 71/223, respectively. There were no significant differences between these values.

When progesterone concentrations were measured in the same samples of medium (Figure 2b), all three gonadotrophin preparations stimulated a dose-dependent rise in progesterone production, but the sensitivity of the progesterone response to IS 71/223 appeared to be less than those produced by rFSH or metrodin. The respective ED_{50} values were: rFSH: 3.1 mIU/ml; metrodin: 2.9 mIU/ml; and IS 71/223: 32 mIU/ml.

Effects of rFSH on granulosa cells from preovulatory follicles

The effects of rFSH (in the absence of IGF-I or HCG) were investigated in four separate experiments using granulosa cell cultures derived from preovulatory follicles which had been obtained either before or just after the start of the LH surge (Table 1, Figures 3 and 4). In three large, pre-LH surge follicles, rFSH produced a clear, dose-related increase in oestradiol production. A typical example is shown in Figure 3.

In one case the cells had been harvested from a follicle after the onset of the LH surge, as judged by blood staining of the follicular fluid.

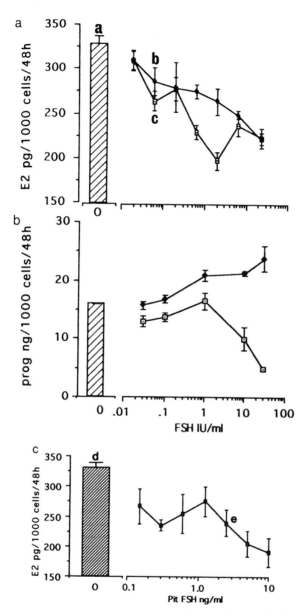

Figure 4 Response to a range of doses of recombinant follicle stimulating hormone (rFSH) (□) and metrodin (♦) (a, b), or pituitary FSH (c) in granulosa cells from a preovulatory follicle after the onset of the luteinizing hormone (LH) surge; (a) oestradiol (b) progesterone. Note inhibition of oestradiol by all FSH preparations (a versus b, $P = 0.006$; a versus c, $P = 0.01$; d versus e, $P = 0.01$) and differential effects on progesterone production. Pituitary FSH had no effect on progesterone production

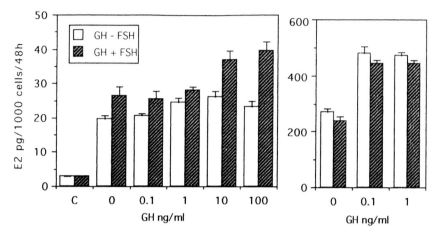

Figure 5 Oestradiol production in response to a range of doses of recombinant growth hormone (GH) with or without pituitary follicle stimulating hormone (FSH) in granulosa cells from a 20 mm follicle prior to luteinizing hormone (LH) surge (left-hand panel) and after onset of LH surge (right-hand panel). Note stimulation of oestradiol production in both cases, despite lack of response to FSH by cells illustrated in right-hand panel

The addition of increasing concentrations of rFSH to these cells progressively inhibited oestradiol accumulation (Figure 4a). Metrodin and the human pituitary FSH had similar inhibitory effects. Interestingly, the three preparations had differential effects on progesterone production by these cells (Figure 4b). Metrodin at higher doses significantly stimulated progesterone accumulation above the control value ($P<0.01$ at 10 IU/ml), whereas rFSH caused inhibition ($P<0.001$ at 10 IU/ml). Pituitary FSH had no effect on progesterone production by these cells.

The oestradiol responses to recombinant growth hormone in the same preovulatory follicles, i.e. just before and after the LH surge, are illustrated in Figure 5. In cells obtained from the follicle removed before the onset of the LH surge, growth hormone induced a small but significant ($P<0.01$ at 10 ng/ml) increase in oestradiol production, which was further augmented by the addition of a fixed dose (5 ng/ml) of human pituitary FSH (Figure 5, left panel). In cultures of cells obtained after exposure to the LH surge, and in contrast to the effects of FSH shown in Figure 4a, growth hormone was able to stimulate oestradiol production ($P<0.001$ at 0.1 ng/ml). There was no additional effect on FSH (Figure 5, right panel).

DISCUSSION

The results presented in this paper demonstrate the efficacy of rFSH (Org 32489) in human granulosa cells and are in keeping with data reported in studies of rat Sertoli cells (Mannaerts *et al.*, 1991). Apart from the intrinsic activity, however, the efficacy of rFSH in the human is mainly determined by its circulating half-life. Clinical phase I studies of rFSH have demonstrated that the elimination half-life of rFSH is comparable to that reported for natural FSH (Mannaerts *et al.*, 1992). The efficacy of rFSH has been illustrated by the reports of successful ovarian stimulation and first established pregnancies (Devroey *et al.*, 1992; Donderwinkel *et al.*, 1992). We have shown that equal amounts of FSH, as judged by the rat in-vivo bioassay of Steelman and Pohley (1953), are able to elicit similar steroid responses in cultured human granulosa cells. The ED_{50} for FSH-stimulated oestradiol production was similar for rFSH, metrodin and IS 71/223. As far as progesterone secretion is concerned, the higher ED_{50} for IS 71/223 when compared with rFSH or metrodin was significant but difficult to explain, since the excess of HCG was added to the cultures at incubation is thought to prevent additional receptor interaction of LH present in IS 71/223. If so, these data could also suggest that minor differences of FSH isohormone profiles may result in a differential regulation of oestrogen and progesterone production.

From an experimental viewpoint, the use of an FSH preparation which is completely free of LH activity enables the investigator to differentiate the effects of FSH from those of LH in cells which are capable of responding to both gonadotrophins i.e. granulosa cells from preovulatory follicles. At supraphysiological doses of FSH there may, however, be some activation of the LH receptor (Mannaerts *et al.*, 1991). In these studies we have shown that granulosa cells taken from preovulatory follicles before the start of the LH surge are capable of secreting oestradiol in a dose-dependent fashion in response to rFSH. These results are consistent with those reported by Yong *et al.* (1992).

An intriguing finding in our study is the apparent inhibitory action of rFSH on oestradiol and progesterone production by granulosa cells obtained from a dominant follicle after the start of the LH surge. A similar observation has recently been reported by Lambert *et al.* (1993), showing that in two of five patients, rFSH inhibited progesterone and oestradiol production by cultured granulosa–lutein cells aspirated at the time of egg collection for in-vitro fertilization (IVF). Granulosa cells cultured from the three other patients were unaffected or slightly stimulated by rFSH, whereas pituitary FSH (IS 83/575) had no effect on oestradiol production, but was stimulatory with respect to progesterone synthesis.

In many species the onset of the LH surge is followed by loss of responsiveness to gonadotrophins, thought to be due, primarily, to down-regulation of gonadotrophin receptors (reviewed by Gore-Langton and Armstrong, 1988). In the human ovary, tissue from pre-ovulatory follicles retains the capacity to aromatize androgens after the LH surge (Edwards et al., 1980) but oestradiol production is low (Le Maire and Marsh, 1975). Therefore, a lack of response to FSH would not have been unexpected, but the observed inhibitory effect of the FSH preparations was surprising. A further explanation is that the granulosa cells with maximal or near maximal aromatase activity would demand an adequate supply of androgen substrate. The concentration of androgen added to the cells (10^{-7} M) may not have been enough to allow maximal oestradiol accumulation. However, one would expect a small rise of oestradiol or no response to FSH rather than a fall in oestradiol concentrations compared with control (no FSH) wells. Furthermore, it is difficult, by this means, to explain the increase in oestradiol in the same cell pool after growth hormone treatment. Pure LH is not currently available, but a similar response to IS 71/223, which contains equal activities of LH and FSH, suggests that LH either has a similar inhibitory action or, at least, is unable to overcome the effect of FSH. These results must be regarded as preliminary and further research will be required to confirm this finding and to elucidate the mechanisms of this action.

We have previously demonstrated a direct gonadotrophic effect of growth hormone on human granulosa cells (Mason et al., 1990b) and interestingly, cells collected after the start of the LH surge retained the response to growth hormone with an increase in oestradiol production. This indicates that it is still possible to stimulate aromatase activity by way of an alternative peptide receptor, possibly via a different pathway. It remains to be determined whether this paradoxical action of FSH has any role in the physiology of the human preovulatory follicle.

ACKNOWLEDGEMENTS

H.D.M. and D.S.W. are supported by the Medical Research Council.

REFERENCES

Alpaugh, K., Indrapichate, K., Abel, J.A., Rimerman, R. and Wimalasena, J. (1990) Purification and characterisation of the human ovarian LH/hCG receptor and comparison of the properties of mammalian LH/hCG receptors. *Biochem. Pharmacol.*, **40**, 2093–2103.

Devroey, P., Van Steirteghem, A., Mannaerts, B. and Coelingh Bennink, H. (1992) Successful in-vitro fertilisation and embryo transfer after treatment with recombinant human FSH. (Letter.) *Lancet*, **339**, May 9, p. 1170.

Donderwinkel, P.F.J., Schoot, D.C., Coelingh Bennink, H.J.T. and Fauser, B.C.J.M. (1992) Pregnancy after induction of ovulation with human recombinant FSH in polycystic ovary syndrome (Letter). *Lancet*, **340**, Oct. 17, p. 983.

Edwards, R.G., Steptoe, P.C., Fowler, R.E. and Baille, J. (1980) Observations on preovulatory human follicles and their aspirates. *Br. J. Obstet. Gynaecol.*, **87**, 769–779.

Erickson, G., Gabriel Garzo, V. and Magoffin, D. (1989) Insulin-like growth factor-I regulates aromatase activity in human granulosa cells and granulosa luteal cells. *J. Clin. Endocrinol. Metab.*, **69**, 716–724.

Gore-Langton, R.E. and Armstrong, D.T. (1988) Follicular steroidogenesis and its control. In Knobil, E. and Neill, J.D. (eds), *The Physiology of Reproduction*. Raven Press, New York, pp. 331–385.

Hillier, S.G. (1991) Cellular basis of follicular endocrine function. In Hillier, S.L. (ed.), *Ovarian Endocrinology*, Blackwell, Oxford, pp. 73–106.

Hsueh, A.J.W., Adashi, E.Y., Jones, P.B.C. and Welsh, T.J. Jr (1984) Hormonal regulation of the differentiation of cultured granulosa cells. *Endocr. Rev.*, **5**, 76–126.

Jia, X., Oikawa, M., Bo, M., Tanaka, T., Ny, T., Biome, I. and Hsueh, A.J.W. (1991) Expression of human luteinising hormone (LH) receptor: Interaction with LH and Chorionic Gonadotrophin from Human but not Enquine, Rat and other species. *Mol. Endocrinol.*, **760**, 759–768.

Lambert, A., Wood, A.M., Hooper, M. and Robertson, W.R. (1993) Recombinant FSH inhibits granulosa lutein cell growth and steroidogenesis in vitro in some patients. *J. Endocrinol.*, **137** (Suppl.), Abstract 169.

LeMaire, W.J. and Marsh, J.M. (1975) Interrelationships between prostaglandins, cyclic AMP and steroids in ovulation. *J. Reprod. Fertil.*, **22**, Suppl., 59–65.

Mannaerts, B., De Leeuw, R., Geelen, J., Van Ravestein, A., Van Wezenbeek, P., Schuurs, A. and Kloosterboer, H. (1991) Comparative in vitro and in vivo studies on the biological characteristics of recombinant human follicle stimulating hormone. *Endocrinology*, **129**, 2623–2630.

Mannaerts, B., Shoham, Z., Schoot, B., Bouchard, P., Harlin, J., Fauser, B., Jacobs, H., Rombout, P. and Coelingh Bennink, H. (1992) Single dose pharmacokinetics and pharmodynamics of recombinant follicle stimulating hormone (Org 32489) in gonadotrophin deficient volunteers. *Fertil. Steril.*, **59**, 108–114.

Mason, H.D., Margara, R., Winston, R.M.L., Beard, R.W., Reed, M.J. and Franks, S. (1990a) Epidermal growth factor inhibits oestradiol production by human granulosa cells from normal and polycystic ovaries. *Clin. Endocrinol.*, **3**, 511–517.

Mason, H.D., Martikainen, H., Beard, R.W., Anyaoku, V. and Franks, S. (1990b) Direct gonadotrophic effects of growth hormone on oestradiol production by human granulosa cells in vitro. *J. Endocrinol.*, **126**, R1–R4.

Mason, H.D., Margara, R., Winston, R.M.L., Seppälä, M., Koistinen, R. and Franks, S. (1993) Insulin-like growth factor I (IGF-I) inhibits production of Insulin-like growth factor binding protein-1 whilst stimulating estradiol secretion in granulosa cells from normal and polycystic ovaries. *J. Clin. Endocrinol. Metab.*, **76**, 1275–1279.

Steelman, S.L. and Pohley, F.M. (1953) Assay of the follicle stimulating hormone based on the augmentation with human chorionic gonadotropin. *Endocrinology*, **53**, 604–616.

Tilly, J.L., Aihara, T., Nishimori, K., Jia, X.-C., Billig, H., Kowalski, K., Perlas, E.A. and Hsueh, A.J.W. (1992) Expression of recombinant human follicle stimulating hormone receptor: Species specific binding, signal transduction, and identification of multiple ovarian messenger ribonucleic acid transcripts. *Endocrinology*, **131**, 799–806.

Yong, E.L., Baird, D.T., Yates, R., Reichert, L.E. and Hillier, S.G. (1992) Hormonal regulation of the growth and steroidogenic function of human granulosa cells. *J. Clin. Endocrinol. Metab.*, **74**, 842–849.

Received June 7, 1993; accepted July 7, 1993

Correspondence: S. Franks, Department of Obstetrics and Gynaecology, Imperial College of Science Technology and Medicine, St Mary's Hospital Medical School, London W2 1PG, UK

3

Circulating bioactive and immunoreactive recombinant human follicle stimulating hormone (Org 32489) after administration to gonadotropin-deficient subjects

T. Matikainen, R. de Leeuw†, B.M.J.L. Mannaerts† and
I. Huhtaniemi**

*Department of Physiology, University of Turku, Turku, Finland, and †Scientific Development Group, NV Organon, Oss, The Netherlands

ABSTRACT

Objective: *To study the bioactivity of recombinant and urinary human FSH after single IM injection into gonadotropin-deficient subjects.*
Design: *Serum FSH levels were measured by immature rat granulosa cell bioassay and immunofluorometric assay. The isohormone distributions of injected FSH materials were analyzed by chromatofocusing. Serum samples were collected before, and 6, 24, and 72 hours after 300 IU of recombinant or urinary FSH.*
Volunteers: *Fifteen gonadotropin-deficient subjects (8 women and 7 men) received recombinant FSH and 8 of them (4 women and 4 men) received an equal dose of urinary FSH.*
Results: *No significant differences were apparent between the bioactive FSH levels after recombinant and urinary FSH treatments (n = 8). The immunoreactive FSH levels at 72 hours after urinary FSH were significantly higher than after recombinant FSH injection with values (median and range) of 3.80 (2.76 to 5.75) IU/L (IRP 78/549) and 3.10 (1.78 to 4.95) IU/L, respectively. There were no significant changes in the bioactive to immunoreactive ratios of FSH within time and between sexes after either recombinant FSH (n = 15) or urinary FSH (n = 8).*

This paper was first published in *Fertility and Sterility*, **61** (1), 62–69 (1994). Reproduced with permission of the publisher, the American Society for Reproductive Medicine (formerly The American Fertility Society) *injected and of the post-treatment serum samples were both higher after recombinant FSH than after urinary FSH injection. Chromatofocusing revealed that injected recombinant FSH contained more activity in the basic fractions than urinary FSH.*

Conclusion: *Recombinant human FSH maintains its biological activity when injected into gonadotropin-deficient subjects. The bioactive to immunoreactive ratio of recombinant FSH was higher than that of urinary FSH indicating that recombinant FSH contains relatively more basic isohormones, and this finding was strengthened by chromatofocusing.*

INTRODUCTION

Gonadotropic hormones, including FSH, exist in the pituitary and circulation in several heterogeneous forms (1–3). This molecular heterogeneity is due to variation in the structures of the carbohydrate moieties, in particular of sialic acid (4–6). These structures have been shown to play an important role in the biochemical and biological characteristics, including receptor binding, in vitro and in vivo bioactivity, and immunogenicity (4, 7–10). Although glycosylation of FSH is not critical for receptor binding, it is important for the receptor-mediated transmembrane signal transduction and circulating half-life (1, 11, 12).

Chinese hamster ovary (CHO) cells, transfected with the human FSH subunit genes, are capable of synthesizing and secreting the intact FSH molecule (13, 14) with identical amino acid composition and oligosaccharide residues closely related to those of the native pituitary hormone found in man. The in vitro and in vivo biological characteristics of recombinant FSH (Org 32489; Organon International bv, Oss, The Netherlands) have been shown to be comparable to those of the natural hormone (15). Previously, the pharmacokinetic properties of recombinant FSH after single intramuscular injection have been studied in hypogonadotropic volunteers by means of a very sensitive immunofluorometric assay (Delfia; Pharmacia, Woerden, The Netherlands) measuring only intact FSH dimers (16). Nevertheless, how long recombinant FSH remains bioactive in the circulation when injected into humans and whether this bioactivity is comparable to that of natural FSH has not been examined. Therefore, in the present study, serum FSH bioactivity was assessed after a single intramuscular injection of 300 IU of recombinant FSH into gonadotropin-deficient subjects and compared with that after urinary human FSH, i.e., Metrodin (Serono, Randolph, MA), injection. The chromatofocusing profiles of both preparations also were determined.

MATERIALS AND METHODS

Subjects and hormone treatments

Eight gonadotropin-deficient women and seven men volunteered for this four-center study. The study was approved by the local Ethical Committees, and written informed consent was obtained from all volunteers. A more detailed description of the subjects has been reported previously (16). Nine subjects had panhypopituitarism, either primary (n = 3) or secondary (n = 6), due to surgical removal of a nonmalignant pituitary tumor. Five volunteers suffered from congenital isolated gonadotropin deficiency, and one volunteer was diagnosed as weight loss-related hypothalamic hypogonadism. With the exception of one man, all subjects had a history of proven normal gonadal function. All were well balanced by substitution treatments in terms of pituitary function, with the exception of gonadotropins. They were in a good health with normal routine laboratory findings. No estrogen/androgen replacement was given during the study. No significant differences between men and women with respect to age (range, 19 to 42 years), height, or weight were found: age and height (mean ± SD) was 36 ± 3 years and 162 ± 12 cm for the women and 31 ± 7 years and 171 ± 13 cm for the men. The mean body weight of the women was 67 ± 14 kg (n = 8) before recombinant FSH injection and 59 ± 13 kg (n = 4) before urinary FSH injection, and the respective values for the men were 62 ± 11 kg (n = 7) and 60 ± 14 kg (n = 4). The body mass index of the women was significantly ($P = 0.02$) higher than that of the men (26 ± 4 versus 21 ± 2).

All subjects received one single intramuscular injection (300 IU; in vivo bioactivity) of recombinant human FSH (Org 32489, CP 90073; 75 IU/ampule) produced by CHO cells, and ≥4 weeks later, eight of the same subjects (four women and four men) received an equal dose of urinary human FSH (Batch 91B14 and 07334109). Based on the outcome of the single dose pharmacokinetic study (16) blood samples were collected just before, and 6 hours (absorption phase), 24 hours (T_{max} of females), and 72 hours (about twice the elimination half-life) after recombinant and urinary FSH injections. The sera were prepared and stored at –20°C until analyzed.

Measurement of bioactive FSH

Serum bioactive FSH was measured by the immature rat in vitro granulosa cell bioassay, as originally described by Jia and Hsueh (17) with some modifications (18, 19). In brief, intact immature (24 to 26 days) female Sprague-Dawley rats were implanted with Silastic capsules releasing diethylstilbestrol (Sigma Chemical Co., St. Louis, MO) to stimulate granulosa cell proliferation. Four days later, the ovaries were dissected out and decapsulated. The follicles were punctured with sterile needles, and granulosa cells were expressed into Medium 199 (GIBCO Ltd., Paisley, Scotland) supplemented with 20 mmol HEPES/L (Sigma), 2 mmol L-glutamine/L (GIBCO), 10^5 IU penicillin/L, 100 mg streptomycin sulfate/L (GIBCO), 30 μg hCG/L (NIH CR-121), 10^{-6} mol 4-androstene-3,17-dione/L (Sigma), 10^{-8} mol DES/L, 0.2 mmol 1-methyl-3-isobutylxanthine/L (Aldrich Chemie, Steinheim, Germany), 1 mg insulin/L (Sigma), 10^{-7} mol P/L (Sigma), 50 mg transferrin/L (Sigma), 10 μg/L recombinant insulin-like growth factor-I (IGF-I, Kabi, Sweden) and 1 μg human recombinant transforming growth factor-β/L (TGF-β, Janssen Biochimica, Geel, Belgium). The cells were cultured (50,000 to 60,000/0.5 mL medium) in 16-mm-diameter 24-well plates.

All serum samples were pretreated with 12% (vol:vol; final concentration) polyethylene glycol (PEG; molecular weight 8,000; Sigma) to remove interfering factors, and a constant serum volume (20 μL) was maintained in all cultures, including the standard (International Reference Preparation [IRP] 78/549) curve, by addition of PEG-pretreated gonadotropin-free serum obtained from women taking oral contraceptive. The immunoreactive FSH level of this serum was 0.17 IU/L, and no stimulation of E_2 production by rat granulosa cells with this serum was observed. After incubation for 72 hours at 37°C in a humidified atmosphere of 5% CO_2 and 95% air, the E_2 content of the medium was measured by RIA (Farmos, Oulunsalo, Finland) after diethylether extraction.

All samples were tested in four concentrations (20, 15, 10, and 5 μL) in triplicate. All samples from each subject collected after either recombinant or urinary FSH injection were measured in the same assay. The interassay and intra-assay coefficients of variation (CVs) calculated using pooled post-menopausal serum diluted to the linear part of the standard curve were 14.2% and 12.6% (n = 10), respectively. The sensitivity of the bioassay was 3.7 ± 1.1 IU/L (mean ± SEM of five assays), defined as the value that is 2 SDs above the mean of the average of 24 zero values per bioassay.

The correlation coefficient of several dilutions of recombinant FSH in the bioassay and immunofluorometric assay was tested before measuring serum samples because varying dose-response characteristics of different in vitro bioassays and immunoassays for FSH have been shown to be responsible for changing ratios of biologically active to immunologically active FSH (20). The correlation of dose-responses of recombinant FSH in rat granulosa cell bioassay and immunofluorometric assay was excellent ($r = 1.00$, $P < 0.001$) in three experiments

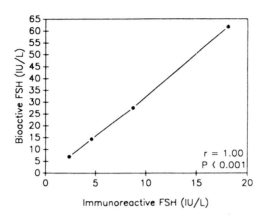

Figure 1 Dose-response characteristics of serially diluted recombinant FSH in rat granulosa cell bioassay (bioactive FSH) and immunofluorometric assay (immunoreactive FSH). The correlation coefficient above the detection limit of FSH bioassay was 1.00 ($P < 0.001$). The figure is representative of one of three similar dose-response experiments

(Figure 1). The bioactive to immunoreactive ratio of recombinant FSH before injection into gonadotropin-deficient subjects was also compared with that of urinary FSH.

Immunofluorometric assay for serum samples

Immunoreactive FSH levels were measured by time-resolved immunofluorometric sandwich assay (Delfia; Pharmacia) as previously described (21, 22). In this assay serial dilution of recombinant and urinary FSH, based on comparable in vivo bioactivities, resulted in dose-related parallel equal responses. The sensitivity of this method is 0.05 IU/L, and the intra-assay and interassay CVs were 4.8% and 4.2%, respectively (22). The FSH standard used was IRP 78/549. The serum reference ranges of FSH, provided by the manufacturer, were 1.0 to 10.5 IU/L for males and 2.4 to 9.3, 3.9 to 13.3, and 0.6 to 8.0 IU/L from women in follicular phase, during ovulation, and in luteal phase, respectively.

Chromatofocusing

Chromatofocusing in the range of pH 6 to 3 was performed on a flow performance liquid chromatography column HR 5/20 (Pharmacia) packed with polybuffer exchanger 94 (Pharmacia) and equilibrated with 0.034 mol L-histidine/L (Aldrich Chemie) adjusted to pH 6.2 with HCl. Before each run the column was eluted with 53 ml polybuffer 74 (Pharmacia) diluted 1:11 (vol:vol) with distilled water and adjusted to pH 3.0 with HCl (elution buffer) and 2 mL 0.034 mol L-histidine containing 100 µg human serum albumin/mL (Bering, Marburg, Germany).

Of both recombinant and urinary FSH, 225 IU FSH was dissolved in 3 mL equilibration buffer (stock solution) and 2 mL of this solution (150 IU) was applied to the column. Subsequently, the column was eluted with the elution buffer. Fractions of 1 mL were collected at a flow rate of 1 mL/min. After 53 fractions, 2 mL of a 2 mol NaCl/L solution were applied to the column and 7 additional fractions were collected. All FSH fractions were desalted by applying each fraction to a PD-10 column (Pharmacia), equilibrated with 12 mL medium$^+$. After elution with 3.5 mL medium$^+$, the collected samples were stored at –20°C until determination of FSH immunoreactivity. Two runs of both FSH preparations were performed.

Immunoreactivity of FSH was measured from individual fractions in a two-site sandwich enzyme immunoassay using beta-directed capturing antibody (monoclonal antibody 4B) and an alpha-directed horseradish peroxidase-labeled detection antibody (monoclonal antibody 116B). This assay recognizes only intact dimers. The assay sensitivity in terms of IS 70/45 was 0.4 IU/L and the intra-assay and interassay CVs were 7% and 8%, respectively. The cross-reactivity with human LH and hCG was <0.001% and <0.001%, respectively.

Data analysis

The data are presented as the median and the range between the minimum and maximum values. Bioactive FSH values below the detection limit are expressed as ND (nondectable) in the text. Statistical analysis within each treatment group was performed by means of the Friedman test. For comparison between treatments only subjects treated with both recombinant and urinary FSH (n = 8) were included. A sign test was used for statistical comparisons of FSH bioactivity and immunoreactivity after both treatments. In addition, the bioactive to immunoreactive ratios were analyzed by the sign rank test. Comparisons between women and men after both treatments were done by Mann–Whitney test. The chromatographic results are expressed as percentages (mean ± SD) of total immunoreactive FSH recovered. $P < 0.05$ was chosen to indicate statistical significance.

RESULTS

The individual levels of women (Figure 2A) and men (Figure 2B) after recombinant human FSH (left panels) and urinary human FSH (right panels) treatments showed great variation with respect to timing and extent. The median values (connected with lines) are shown in Figure 2, and the respective bioactive to immunoreactive ratios after both treatments are presented in Table 1. A good correlation between FSH bioactivity and immunoreactivity was found ($r = -0.84$, $P = 0.001$) after recombinant FSH treatment as well as a negative association between the bioactive FSH level and body weight ($r = 0.6$ for women and $r = -0.8$ for men). At 6 hours after injection, the bioactive and immunoreactive FSH levels in men were significantly higher than those in women. The respective bioactive levels for men and women were 25.5 (14.5 to 92.3) IU/L ($P = 0.046$ versus in women) and 9.9 (ND to 27.8) IU/L, and those of immunoreactive FSH levels were 7.2 (3.1 to 16.8) IU/L ($P = 0.0053$ versus women) and 2.7 (1.3 to 5.3) IU/L, respectively. Comparable findings were made after urinary FSH treatment.

The comparisons between recombinant and urinary FSH treatments were performed only between subjects having received both preparations (n = 8). The bioactive FSH levels after recombinant FSH treatment tended to be higher than those after urinary FSH treatment, although this difference was not statistically significant. The immunoreactive FSH level showed an opposite tendency, but only at 72 hours after urinary FSH injection: the immunoreactive FSH levels were significantly higher than those after recombinant FSH injection. The respective values were 3.80 (2.76 to 5.75) IU/L and 3.10 (1.78 to 4.95) IU/L ($P = 0.016$).

Although the bioactive to immunoreactive ratio after urinary FSH injection tended to decrease with time, no significant changes in the bioactive to immunoreactive ratios after either recombinant FSH (n = 15) or urinary FSH (n = 8) treatments were found within time. In addition, there was no significant difference in that parameter between women and men (Table 1). However, in all after-treatment samples the bioactive to immunoreactive ratio was significantly higher after recombinant FSH treatment than after urinary FSH treatment (Figure 3). The respective FSH ratios (median and range of both sexes) at 6, 24, and 72 hours were 3.8 (1.7 to 8.2) ($P = 0.0078$ versus urinary FSH), 3.6 (1.7 to 5.8) ($P = 0.0078$), and 5.4 (ND to 9.7) ($P = 0.031$) after recombinant FSH (n = 8) injection and 2.0 (0.47 to 4.73), 2.0 (ND to 2.73), and 0.9 (ND to 6.50) after urinary FSH (n = 8) treatment (Figure 3).

When the injected recombinant and urinary FSH solutions were analyzed in the same bioassay (n = 3), the median bioactive to immunoreactive ratio of recombinant FSH was 2.7-fold higher than that of urinary FSH ($P = 0.046$). Chromatofocusing of the material injected

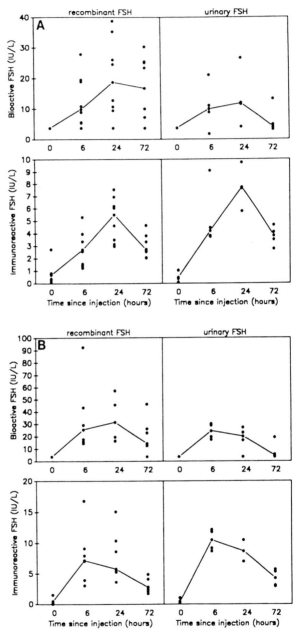

Figure 2 Serum bioactive (upper panels) and immunoreactive (lower panels) FSH values (scatter plots) and medians (connected with lines) after intramuscular injection of 300 IU of recombinant (left panels) and urinary (right panels) human FSH in gonadotropin-deficient women (A) and men (B). The bioactive FSH values below detection limit are expressed as the detection limit

Table 1 Serum bioactive to immunoreactive ratios of FSH after 300 IU of recombinant and urinary FSH in women and men*

Time after injection	Recombinant FSH†	Urinary FSH‡
Women		
0 h	ND§	ND
6 h	3.4 (ND to 14.5)	1.8 (0.5 to 4.7)
24 h	3.7 (ND to 7.7)	1.6 (0.7 to 2.7)
72 h	4.6 (ND to 9.7)	0.9 (ND to 3.8)
Men		
0 h	ND	ND
6 h	4.1 (2.2 to 5.5)	2.4 (1.4 to 3.5)
24 h	4.4 (3.1 to 5.6)	2.5 (ND to 2.7)
72 h	5.2 (ND to 21.0)	1.1 (ND to 6.4)

*Values are medians between the minimum and maximum values with ranges in parentheses.
†Women, n = 8; men, n = 7.
‡Women, n = 4; men, n = 4.
§ND, below the detection limit in the particular FSH bioassay.

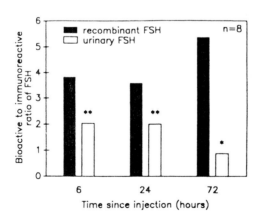

Figure 3 The bioactive to immunoreactive ratios of FSH after 300 IU of recombinant human FSH (black bars; n = 8) and urinary human FSH (white bars; n = 8). *$P < 0.05$, **$P < 0.01$ versus after recombinant FSH treatment

Table 2 Isohormone distributions of recombinant and urinary FSH after chromatofocusing

	Distribution of immunoreactive FSH*	
pH range	Recombinant FSH (%)	Urinary FSH (%)
6.00 to 5.30	2.1 ± 0.1	0.0 ± 0.0
5.29 to 4.70	17.2 ± 2.1	5.8 ± 0.3
4.69 to 4.10	58.7 ± 6.1	48.6 ± 7.2
4.09 to 3.60	18.7 ± 3.6	34.4 ± 4.7
3.59 to 3.00	2.7 ± 0.3	6.5 ± 1.0
<3.00	0.8 ± 0.0	4.7 ± 1.1
Recovery	85.9 ± 7.1	89.9 ± 2.5

*Values are mean ± SD of two separate runs of both FSH preparations.

revealed that recombinant FSH contains more activity in the basic fractions than urinary FSH (Table 2), which finding is well in agreement with the difference in the bioactive to immunoreactive ratios.

DISCUSSION

In the present study we have for the first time shown that circulating recombinant FSH is biologically active at least during the 72-hour test period after single intramuscular injection. No change in the bioactive to immunoreactive ratio of recombinant FSH was found between the 6, 24, and 72 hour samples analyzed in these 15 gonadotropin-deficient subjects. In accordance, a good correlation ($r = 0.84$, $P = 0.001$) between bioactive and immunoreactive FSH levels in serum samples was demonstrated up to 72 hours after recombinant FSH, which indicates that the circulating amounts of immunoreactive recombinant FSH represent well the bioactivity at the target cell level. For the interpretation of clinical pharmacodynamic studies this finding is of great importance.

When the bioactive to immunoreactive ratio was measured after urinary FSH treatment, it tended to decrease with time, although the decrease was not statistically significant. In earlier studies, serum bioactive FSH levels after urinary FSH injections were shown to decrease faster than those of immunoreactive levels, and the half-life of bioactive FSH was shown to be much shorter than that of immunoreactive FSH (23). In all serum samples drawn later than 36 hours after intramuscular injection of 450 IU of urinary FSH, bioactive FSH was not detectable. The difference between these data (23) and the present data may be due to different assay sensitivity, which was higher in our study. We also were able to detect bioactivities in most of the samples 72 hours after injections of 300 IU of both FSH preparations.

Although the bioactivity of the recombinant FSH samples tended to be higher than those of urinary FSH and the immunoreactivities displayed an opposite trend, no significant differences between the two hormone preparations were observed in these parameters except in immunoreactive levels at 72 hours. The minor differences in the bioactivities and immunoreactivities were reflected by greater differences in the bioactive to immunoreactive ratios. In all after-treatment samples, the ratio of recombinant FSH was significantly higher than that of urinary FSH. A comparable difference (approximately 2.7-fold) in the ratios was also found between the injection solution of recombinant FSH and urinary FSH. This finding suggests that in comparison to urinary FSH, recombinant FSH contains more basic isoforms both before and after injection. The results after chromatofocusing strongly support this finding, because recombinant FSH contained significantly more activity in basic fractions than urinary FSH. However, it remains to be investigated whether batch-to-batch differences of each gonadotropin preparation contribute to these observed differences.

It previously has been shown by chromatofocusing studies that during the midfollicular phase of the normal menstrual cycle relatively more basic, and thus in vitro more bioactive, isoforms are present than during luteal or follicular phase (24). Whether the observed differences in the bioactive to immunoreactive ratios and isohormone distributions of recombinant and urinary FSH have any clinical relevance under steady state conditions remains to be examined in extensive group comparative clinical studies. Because of a decrease in the bioactive to immunoreactive ratio of urinary FSH, the difference in that ratio after recombinant FSH and urinary FSH treatment tended to increase, although not significantly, indicating that there might be a shift in the isohormone composition during the clearance of urinary FSH, whereas this is less obvious for recombinant FSH.

It only recently has been reported that recombinant FSH is absorbed from its intramuscular depot to a higher rate and extent in men than in women (16). It has also been suggested that there is a linear relationship between body weight and serum immunoreactive FSH level (16). Similar relationship was also found in bioactive FSH levels when women and men were compared and when body weight was correlated with bioactive FSH level. Obviously, part of the intersubject variability is due to body weight differences. However, in earlier studies with human menopausal gonadotropins, significant differences were also found in intraindividual responses of patients exposed to the same dose of FSH (25) and, moreover, these differences were independent of the FSH preparation used. These findings strongly suggested individual differences in the metabolism of the gonadotropins administered (25). No differences in the bioactive to immunoreactive ratio of FSH was found between women and men, indicating that after single injection the clearance of the different isohormones is similar in both sexes.

In conclusion, recombinant FSH remained biologically active when injected into gonadotropin-deficient subjects, and the in vitro bioactivity of FSH was similar to that after urinary human FSH injection, indicating similar effectiveness at the target cell level. However, the bioactive to immunoreactive ratio of recombinant FSH was higher than that of urinary FSH and recombinant FSH contained significantly more activity in the basic fraction. These findings suggest that recombinant FSH resembles more closely the previously reported FSH isohormone composition during the midfollicular phase of the menstrual cycle.

ACKNOWLEDGEMENTS

We thank the clinical investigators, Howard Jacobs, M.D., Cobbold Laboratories, Middlesex Hospital, London, United Kingdom; Philip Bouchard, M.D., Service d'Endocrinologie et des Maladies de la Reproduction, Hopital Bicêtre, Kremlin Bicêtre, France; Bart Fauser, M.D., Department of Obstetrics and Gynaecology, Dijkzigt Hospital Rotterdam, Rotterdam, The Netherlands; and Jonas Harlin, M.D., Department of Obstetrics and Gynaecology, Karolinska Hospital, Stockholm, Sweden.

The skillful technical assistance of Ms. Tarja Laiho, Ms. Anne-Mari Fredriksson, and Ms. Lenita Timmer is gratefully acknowledged. Mr. Unto Alapiessa, M.Sc. and Ms. Tiina Töyrylä are also gratefully acknowledged for their kind assistance during this project.

REFERENCES

1. Ulloa-Aguirre A, Cravioto A, Damian-Matsumura P, Jimenez M, Zambrano E, Diaz-Sanches V. Biological characterization of the naturally occurring analogues of intrapituitary human follicle-stimulating hormone. Hum Reprod 1992;7:23–30.
2. Wide L. The regulation of metabolic clearance rate of human FSH in mice by variation of the molecular structure of the hormone. Acta Endocrinol (Copenh) 1986;112:336–44.

3. Stanton PG, Robertson DM, Burgon PG, Schmauk-White B, Hearn MTW. Isolation and physicochemical characterization of human follicle-stimulating hormone isoforms. Endocrinology 1992;130:2820–32.
4. Ulloa-Aguirre A, Espinoza R, Damian Matsumura P, Chappel SC. Immunological and biological potencies of different molecular species of gonadotropins. Hum Reprod 1988;3:491–501.
5. Green ED, Baenziger JU. Asparagine-linked oligosaccharides of lutropin, follitropin, and thyrotropin. I. Structural elucidation of the sulphated and sialylated oligosaccharides on bovine, ovine and human pituitary glycoprotein hormones. J Biol Chem 1988;263:25–35.
6. Green ED, Baenziger JU. Asparagine-linked oligosaccharides of lutropin, follitropin, and thyrotropin. II. Distributions of sulphated and sialylated oligosaccharides on bovine, ovine and human pituitary glycoprotein hormones. J Biol Chem 1988;263:36–44.
7. Keel BA, Grotjan HE, editors. Microheterogeneity of the glycoprotein hormones. Boca Raton (FL): CRC Press, 1989:149–84.
8. Chappel SC, Ulloa-Aquirre A, Coutifaris C. Biosynthesis and secretion of follicle-stimulating hormone. Endocr Rev 1983;4:179–211.
9. Pierce JG, Parsons TF. Glycoprotein hormones: structure and function. Annu Rev Biochem 1981;50:465–95.
10. Cerpa-Poljak A, Bishop LA, Hort YJ, Chin CKH, DeKroon R, Mahler SM, et al. Isoelectric charge of recombinant human follicle-stimulating hormone isoforms determines receptor affinity and in vitro bioactivity. Endocrinology 1993;132:351–6.
11. Sairam MR, Bhargavi GN. A role of glycosylation of the α subunit in transduction of biological signal in glycoprotein hormones. Science 1985;229:65–7.
12. Sairam MR. Protein glycosylation and receptor-ligand interactions. In: Conn PM, editor. The receptors. Vol. II. New York: Academic Press, 1985:307–40.
13. Keene JL, Matzuk MM, Otani T, Fauser BCJM, Galway B, Hsueh AJW, et al. Expression of biologically active human follitropin in Chinese hamster ovary cells. J Biol Chem 1989;264:4769–75.
14. Van Wezenbeek P, Draaijer J, van Meel F, Olijve W. Recombinant follicle-stimulating hormone I. Construction, selection and characterization of a cell line. In: Crommelin DJA, Schellekens H, editors. From clone to clinic, developments in biotherapy. Vol. 1. Dordrecht, The Netherlands: Kluwer, 1990:245–51.
15. Mannaerts B, De Leeuw R, Geelen J, Van Ravestein A, Van Wezenbeek P, Schuurs A, et al. Comparative in vitro and in vivo studies on the biological characteristics of recombinant human follicle-stimulating hormone. Endocrinology 1991;129:2623–30.
16. Mannaerts B, Shoham Z, Schoot D, Bouchard P, Harlin J, Fauser B, et al. Single dose pharmacokinetics and pharmacodynamics of recombinant human follicle-stimulating hormone (Org 32489) in gonadotropin-deficient volunteers. Fertil Steril 1993;59: 108–14.
17. Jia X-C, Hsueh AJW. Granulosa cell aromatase bioassay for follicle-stimulating hormone: validation and application of the method. Endocrinology 1986;119:1570–7.

18. Reddi K, Wickings EJ, McNeilly AS, Baird DT, Hillier SG. Circulating bioactive follicle stimulating hormone and immunoreactive inhibin levels during the normal human menstrual cycle. Clin Endocrinol (Oxf) 1990;33:547–57.
19. Matikainen T, Ding Y-Q, Vergara M, Huhtaniemi I, Couzinet B, Schaison G. Differing responses of plasma bioactive and immunoreactive FSH and LH to GnRH antagonist and agonist treatments in postmenopausal women. J Clin Endocrinol Metab 1992;75:820–5.
20. Jockenhövel F, Khan SA, Nieschlag E. Varying dose-response characteristics of different immunoassays and an in-vitro bioassay for FSH are responsible for changing ratios of biologically active to immunologically active FSH. J Endocrinol 1990;127:523–32.
21. Lövgren T, Hemmilä I, Pettersson K, Eskola JU, Bertoft E. Determination of hormones by time-resolved fluoroimmunoassay. Talanta 1984;31:909–16.
22. Jaakkola T, Ding Y-Q, Kellokumpu-Lehtinen P, Valavaara R, Martikainen H, Tapanainen J, et al. The ratios of serum bioactive/immunoreactive luteinizing hormone and follicle-stimulating hormone in various clinical conditions with increased and decreased gonadotropin secretion: re-evaluation by a highly sensitive immunometric assay. J Clin Endocrinol Metab 1990;70:1496–505.
23. Jockenhövel F, Fingscheidt U, Khan SA, Behre HM, Nieschlag E. Bio and immuno-activity of FSH in serum after intramuscular injection of highly purified urinary human FSH in normal men. Clin Endocrinol (Oxf) 1990;33:573–84.
24. Padmanabhan V, Land LL, Sonstein J, Kelch RP, Beitins IZ. Modulation of serum follicle-stimulating hormone bioactivity and isoform distribution by estrogenic steroids in normal women and in gonadal dysgenesis. J Clin Endocrinol Metab 1988;67:465–73.
25. Diczfalusy E, Harlin J. Clinical-pharmacological studies on human menopausal gonadotropin. Hum Reprod 1988;3:21–7.

Received May 7; revised and accepted September 13, 1993

Correspondence: Ilpo Huhtaniemi, M.D., Department of Physiology, University of Turku, Kiinamyllynkatu 10, FIN-20520 Turku, Finland

4

Folliculogenesis in hypophysectomized rats after treatment with recombinant human follicle-stimulating hormone

B.M.J.L. Mannaerts*, J. Uilenbroek[†], P. Schot* and R. de Leeuw*

*Scientific Development Group, NV Organon, 5340 BH Oss, The Netherlands, and [†]Department of Endocrinology and Reproduction, Erasmus University, Rotterdam, The Netherlands

ABSTRACT

To examine the role of FSH and LH in follicular growth and atresia, immature hypophysectomized (hypox) rats were treated twice daily for four days with a total dose either of 2.5 to 40 IU recombinant human FSH (recFSH; Org 32489) or of 8 IU recFSH supplemented with 0.2 to 5 IU hCG.

RecFSH alone caused dose-dependent increases in ovarian weight and intraovarian estradiol (E_2) but was unable to elevate circulating E_2 levels. The number of antral follicles was also increased in a recFSH dose-dependent manner, and a gradual shift of small antral follicles to large preovulatory follicles was noted. The latter ovulated after a single bolus injection of 10 IU hCG. In comparison with follicles from hypox vehicle-treated animals, these follicles showed a diminished incidence of atresia, especially in the smallest size class of antral follicles. A total dose of ≥10 IU recFSH increased uterine weight accompanied by endometrium proliferation.

When 8 IU recFSH was supplemented with 0.2 to 5 IU hCG, ovarian weight was augmented in an hCG dose-dependent fashion, but no further increases in total number of antral follicles were noted except with the highest hCG dose given. Nevertheless, addition of relatively low doses

This paper was first published in *Biology of Reproduction*, **51**, 72–81 (1994). Reproduced by permission of The Society for the Study of Reproduction *of hCG caused considerable shifts of small follicles to large, preovulatory follicles. Furthermore, supplementation with hCG, especially low dosages of hCG (0.2 and 0.5 IU), reduced the incidence of atresia in antral follicles of all size classes.*

These data suggest that in the complete absence of LH activity, recFSH induces follicular growth up to the stage of mature preovulatory follicles and induces ovarian estradiol production and endometrium proliferation. The addition of small amounts of LH activity increases the percentage of healthy follicles.

INTRODUCTION

The relative contributions of FSH and LH in the control of folliculogenesis have been under investigation for many years; and several models for follicular selection and development, resulting in single or multiple ovulation, have been proposed [1–3]. The conversion of primordial into primary follicles is thought to be gonadotropin-independent, since this process continues normally after hypophysectomy. The further development of growing follicles up to the antral stage can occur in the absence of gonadotropins, although quantitatively this process will be strongly inhibited. Whenever a follicle reaches the antral stage and the level of FSH exceeds a certain threshold value, the fol-licle continues its development to the preovulatory stage. However, if the antral stage is reached and FSH levels are insufficient, follicles become atretic. The total number of selected follicles would depend on the (species-dependent) degree of synchrony by which follicular growth is initiated as well as the time period during which the level of FSH remains above this threshold value.

The exact role of LH during folliculogenesis is less well understood, since granulosa cells of developing follicles acquire their LH receptors only in the antral stage in response to FSH and estradiol (E_2) [4]. Only recently, it has been demonstrated that recombinant human FSH (recFSH), devoid of LH activity, stimulates multiple follicular growth up to the preovulatory stage in immature, hypophysectomized (hypox) rats, whereas circulating levels of E_2 remain low at baseline [5]. The latter finding is in agreement with the two-cell, two-gonadotropin theory holding that both FSH and LH activity are required for estrogen biosynthesis [4]. Studies in gonadotropin-deficient women using recFSH or urinary FSH have confirmed that FSH administered alone can induce follicular growth but that small amounts of LH are essential for adequate steroidogenesis and subsequent endometrial proliferation [6–8]. On the other hand, excessive amounts of LH activity are thought to exert detrimental effects on the maturation of ovulatory follicles, causing atresia and premature resumption of meiosis [1].

The current study was undertaken to gain further knowledge about the role of FSH and LH activity in follicular growth and atresia and simultaneous uterine development. For this purpose, immature hypox rats were treated with recFSH or with recFSH supplemented with hCG. Effects on ovaries were evaluated by assessment of ovarian weight, ovarian E_2 and androstenedione production, and the number of healthy and atretic antral follicles of the various size classes [9]. In addition the uterus was weighed and histologically examined.

MATERIALS AND METHODS

Animals

Immature female Wistar rats (45–50 g, 21 days old) were purchased from Harlan CPB (Zeist, The Netherlands) and housed in a temperature-controlled room, at 21°C before and 25°C after hypophysectomy, with a light cycle of 14L:10D. The animals had free access to standard pelleted food and tap water.

Gonadotropins

Highly purified (>99%) lyophilised recFSH (Org 32489, batch 65) was supplied by Diosynth (Oss, The Netherlands), and hCG (Pregnyl, batch 05-2135) was supplied by NV Organon (Oss, The Netherlands). The specific in vivo bioactivity of the recFSH preparation was 13 100 (12 100–14 300) IU/mg protein [5]. The in vivo bioactivity of the hCG preparation was 520 IU/ampule. For injection, gonadotropins were dissolved in a buffer (pH 7.2) consisting of 43.7 mM NaH_2PO_4, 109.7 mM Na_2HPO_4, 0.1% methylhydroxybenzoate, and 0.1% gelatin.

Experiments

The procedure for these experiments has been described previously [5]. Animals were hypophysectomized at 22 days of age; four days later, if animals had not gained weight, treatment was started by means of twice daily s.c. injections of recFSH (total doses: 2.5, 5, 10, 20, 40 IU) or recFSH supplemented with hCG (total doses: 0.2, 0.5, 2, 5 IU). In experiments with hCG supplementation, a total sub-maximal dose of 8 IU recFSH was used. Control animals were treated with vehicle solution only or with hCG only (total dose, 5 IU). After four days of treatment, 18 h after the last injection, animals were administered diethylether anesthesia and were exsanguinated by drawing blood from the abdominal aorta. Animals with pituitary remnants in the sella turcica were excluded. Ovaries and uterus were dissected out and weighed. From each animal, one ovary was fixed in Bouin's fluid for histological examination and one ovary was frozen at −80°C until determination of levels of E_2 and androstenedione. Uteri of animals treated with vehicle only or with 40 IU recFSH were also fixed in Bouin's fluid for histological examination. In one of the experiments described above, animals treated with 20 or 40 IU recFSH only were given a bolus injection of 10 IU hCG to induce ovulation. HCG was administered simultaneously with the last injection of recFSH. Eighteen hours thereafter, tubes were inspected for the presence of oocytes. If animals had ovulated, ovaries were examined histologically for the presence of CL.

Steroid assessments

Intraovarian and plasma E_2 was measured in a 17β–E_2 kit (detection limit 10 pg/ml; ICN Biomedicals, Inc. Carson, CA), and intraovarian androstenedione was measured in an androstenedione kit (detection limit 40 pg/ml; ICN Biomedicals).

The intra- and interassay coefficients of variation were 6.4% (higher detection limit) to 10.6% (lower detection limit) and 5.9% (higher detection limit) to 11.9% (lower detection limit) for E_2 and <5% and <6% for androstenedione, respectively. In the E_2 assay, the cross-reactivity with estrone was 20%; in the androstenedione assay, the cross-reactivity with androsterone was 0.03%.

Before analysis, plasma samples were extracted with methanol using octadecyl columns (Baker, Deventer, The Netherlands). After evaporation to dryness, the residues were dissolved in assay buffer. During this step, samples were concentrated at maximum five times, increasing the sensitivity of the E_2 assay from approximately 10 to 2 pg/ml.

For the measurement of intraovarian E_2 and androstenedione, ovaries were homogenised and extracted three times with 1 ml of methanol. After evaporation to dryness, the ovarian residues were dissolved in 1 ml charcoal-treated human serum with E_2 and androstenedione levels below the detection limit of the respective assay. The tissue extracts were assayed after methanol extraction using octadecyl columns. During extraction, samples were concentrated at maximum five times, increasing the sensitivity of the E_2 and androstenedione assay from approximately 10 to 2 pg/ml and from 40 to 8 pg/ml. respectively.

Histology

For histological examination, fixed ovaries and uterine material were embedded in paraffin, and serial sections (6 to 10 μm) were stained with hematoxylin and eosin. Differential follicle counts were made according to the method described by Osman [9]. In one ovary from each animal, follicles of a mean diameter >275 μm were counted. Five follicle size classes were distinguished: class 1 (275–350 μm), class 2 (351–400 μm), class 3 (401–450 μm), class 4 (451–575 μm), and class 5 (≥576 μm). Follicles of these sizes were all antral follicles. The mean follicle diameter was calculated from the two perpendicular diameters in the section containing the oocyte nucleolus. Degenerative changes detectable by light microscopy were used as criteria for atresia in each counted follicle. In principle, two stages of atresia were distinguished, i.e., early and late atresia. Follicles with early atresia included those in which the granulosa cell wall showed cell shrinkage and only a few pyknotic cells were present (stage Ia [9]), as well as those in which the whole granulosa cell wall was affected by degeneration and pyknotic cells were present in the periphery of the antrum (stage Ib [9]). Follicles with late atresia contained oocytes showing resumption of meiosis – though still surrounded by granulosa cells (stage IIa [9]), or "naked" oocytes showing resumption of meiosis (stage IIb [9])

Statistical analysis

Statistical analysis of responses was performed according to a randomized design, and significance was defined as $p<0.05$. Ovarian and uterus weight, ovarian E_2, and plasma E_2 were expressed as geometric means with SEM and were compared, after log transformation of the original data, by a one-way variance analysis with pairwise t-tests (for comparison of unknowns with control). Statistical analysis of follicle counts, which were expressed as means with SEM, was performed by means of Wilcoxon's test.

RESULTS

RecFSH alone

The effect of recFSH on ovarian weight, uterine weight, ovarian E_2, and plasma E_2 in immature, hypox rats is presented in Table 1. Total dosages of 2.5, 5, 10, 20, and 40 IU recFSH induced dose-dependent increases in ovarian weight from 7.6±0.7 mg in vehicle-treated animals (controls) to 35.3±2.4 mg in animals treated with 40 IU recFSH. Com-

Table 1 Effect of recFSH in immature hypophysectomized rats treated twice daily for 4 days

Treatment total dose (IU)	N^a	Ovarian weight (mg)	Ovarian estradiol (pg/ovary)	Plasma estradiol (pg/ml)	Uterine weight (mg)
0	6	7.6 ± 0.7	4.2 ± 0.5	4.0 ± 1.1	15.8 ± 0.8
2.5	5	11.0 ± 1.2*	7.1 ± 2.7	1.9 ± 0.4	18.3 ± 3.5
5	5	12.8 ± 1.6*	13.3 ± 3.9*	2.8 ± 1.0	17.9 ± 2.6
10	5	28.8 ± 3.1*	24.8 ± 7.0*	2.5 ± 0.4	34.2 ± 15.7*
20	4	28.2 ± 3.2*	32.3 ± 7.4*	1.9 ± 0.3	50.4 ± 14.8*
40	6	35.3 ± 2.4*	72.0 ± 16.9*	4.2 ± 1.4	68.1 ± 11.6*

[a]N represents the number of animals per treatment group.
*Significantly ($p<0.05$) increased in comparison to vehicle treatment only.

pared to the value for controls, a significant ($p<0.05$) increase was noted with the lowest dose of 2.5 IU recFSH, while a maximal response was reached at 10 IU recFSH. In contrast to circulating E_2 levels, which remained low at baseline level, intraovarian E_2 and uterine weight increased with the dose of recFSH given. Total dosages of 0 to 40 IU recFSH induced increases in intraovarian E_2 from 4.2 ± 0.5 pg/ovary (control) to 72.0 ± 16.9 pg/ovary and in uterine weight from 15.8 ± 0.8 mg (control) to 68.1 ± 11.6 mg. In comparison to controls, significant ($p<0.05$) increases were noted at a total dose of ≥5 IU recFSH for ovarian E_2 and at a total dose of ≥10 IU for uterine weight. Levels of ovarian E_2 induced by the highest dose of recFSH were comparable to those of intact, immature animals (72.0 ± 16.9 and 79.4 ± 6.3 pg/ovary, respectively). In contrast, ovarian androstenedione was undetectable (<8 pg/ovary) both in intact animals and in recFSH-treated hypox animals.

The total number of healthy and atretic antral follicles and their distribution over the various size classes are depicted in Table 2 and Figure 1, respectively. Typical histological illustrations of ovarian and uterine sections are presented in Figure 3.

The total number of antral follicles was increased in a dose-dependent manner from 11 ± 4 per ovary in controls to 80 ± 7 per ovary in animals treated with 40 IU recFSH. As with the increases in ovarian weight, a significant ($p<0.05$) rise in number of follicles was induced by doses ≥2.5 IU recFSH and maximal response was reached at 10 IU recFSH (Table 2). Antral follicles of controls were 69% atretic (Table 2, Figure 3, A and B). The incidence of follicular atresia decreased due to recFSH treatment from 69% in controls to 31% in animals treated with

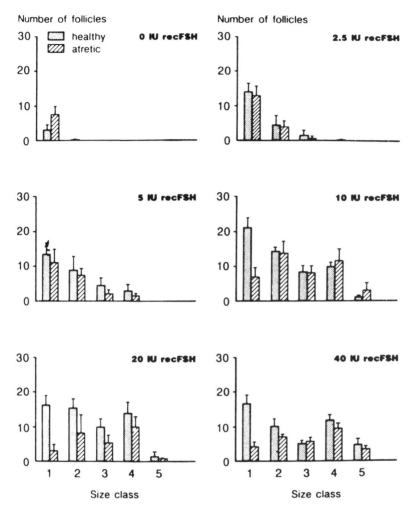

Figure 1 Number of healthy and atretic antral follicles in various size classes (mean diameter class 1:275–350; class 2:351–400; class 3:401–450; class 4:451–575; class 5: ≥576 µm) present in one ovary after treatment of immature, hypox rats with 0 to 40 IU recFSH. "Other" follicles with loosely arranged granulosa cells (40 IU recFSH, size classes 1 to 5) were included as atretic follicles

20 IU recFSH. This decrease in atresia was most apparent and most dependent on the dose in size class 1 follicles (Figure 1). Treatment with increasing doses of recFSH caused a gradual shift in follicle counts from size class 1 (0 IU) via size classes 2 and 3 (2.5 IU) to size classes 4 and 5 (≥5 IU).

After treatment with 40 IU recFSH, 39% of all antral follicles were classified as atretic, i.e., 6% as early and late atretic and 33% as "other"

Table 2 Effect of recFSH alone on numbers of healthy and atretic follicles in immature hypophysectomized rats

Total dose (IU) recFSH	N^a	Total number of follicles ($>275\mu m$)	Number of atretic follicles ($275\mu m$)			Percentage of atretic follicles ($>275\mu m$)
			Early atretic[b]	Late atretic[c]	Other[d]	
0	6	11 ± 4	6.5 ± 2.0	1.0 ± 0.5	–	69 ± 15
2.5	5	36 ± 4*	13.2 ± 2.1	3.0 ± 1.2	–	45 ± 8
5	4	52 ± 12*	17.8 ± 3.8	4.3 ± 1.7	–	44 ± 9
10	5	99 ± 6*	35.6 ± 2.7	8.0 ± 3.3	–	44 ± 3
20	4	85 ± 14*	27.0 ± 11.0	0.5 ± 0.5	–	31 ± 9
40	6	80 ± 7*	0.5 ± 0.2	3.8 ± 1.7	26 ± 3	39 ± 2

[a] N represents the number of animals per treatment group.
[b] Early atretic: stage 1a and 1b.
[c] Late atretic: stage 2a and 2b.
[d] Other: follicles with loosely arranged granulosa cells.
Significantly ($p < 0.05$) increased in comparison to vehicle treatment only.

(see Table 2). These latter follicles exhibited loosely arranged granulosa cells around the oocyte and an antral layer without pyknosis and a large number of mitotic figures (Figure 3, C and D). The appearance of these follicles was very similar to that seen in proestrous animals several hours after the LH surge, but in contrast, no germinal vesicle breakdown was observed and the interstitium had a somewhat atrophic appearance. Although these follicles were not included in the classification of Osman [9], they were regarded in the present study as atretic follicles, especially since continuation of treatment with this highest dose of recFSH for another four days induced both early and late atretic follicles with pyknosis and macrophage invasion (data not shown).

When hypox animals were treated for four days with recFSH only, no CL were observed. The subsequent administration of 10 IU hCG to animals treated with 20 or 40 IU recFSH resulted in ovulation in 7 of 8 and 8 of 8 animals, respectively. The median (range) number of CL was 3 (0–28) and 6 (0–26) per ovary, respectively. In addition to CL, large follicles with loosely arranged granulosa cells and germinal vesicle breakdown were present, but large healthy (size class 5) follicles were absent.

Histological examination of uterine endothelium originating from animals treated with vehicle only or with 40 IU recFSH revealed that the height and number of epithelial cells and the folding of the endometrial layer were markedly increased (Figure 3, E and F). Although

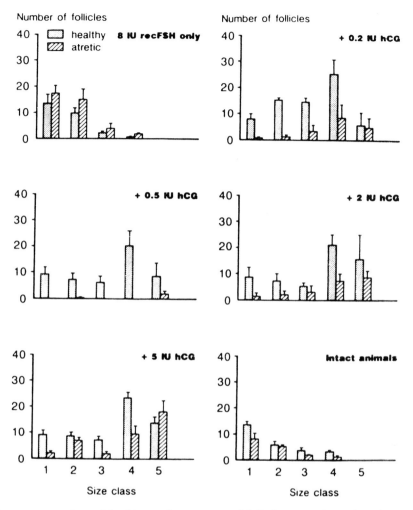

Figure 2 Number of healthy and atretic antral follicles in various size classes (as specified in legend to Figure 1) present in one ovary after treatment of immature, hypox rats with 8 IU recFSH supplemented with 0 to 5 IU hCG. "Other" follicles with loosely arranged granulosa cells (8 IU recFSH with 2 or 5 IU hCG; size classes 4 to 5) were included as atretic follicles

the number of epithelial cells per micrometer was unchanged, the number of cells lining the uterine cavity was increased fourfold (data not shown). As seen in Figure 3, E and F, the height of the epithelial glandular cells in the endometrial stroma and the thickness of the latter layer were increased after treatment with 40 IU recFSH.

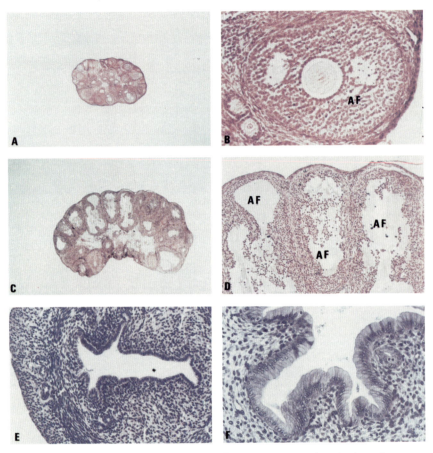

Figure 3 A and B Sections of ovaries after treatment with vehicle solution at magnification × 2.5 and × 25, respectively. Only a limited number of small antral follicles (size class 1), mainly early atretic, are perceptible.

C and D Sections of ovaries after treatment with 40 IU recFSH at magnification × 2.5 and × 10, respectively. Atretic antral follicles with dispersion of granulosa cells, a thin granulosa cell layer and an atrophic interstitium are apparent.

E and F Uterine sections after treatment with vehicle only and after treatment with 40 IU recFSH at magnification × 25 and × 25, respectively. Folding of the endometrial layer, height and number of epithelial cells, glandular cells and endometrial stroma are clearly increased due to recFSH treatment

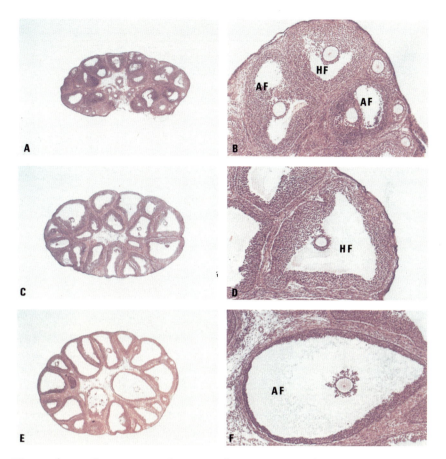

Figure 4 A and B Sections of ovaries after treatment with 8 IU recFSH at magnification × 2.5 and × 10, respectively. Antral follicles of size classes 1 to 4 are present. The highest magnification shows one healthy follicle (HF) and two atretic follicles (AF) of size class 2.

C and D Sections of ovaries after treatment with 8 IU recFSH and 0.2 IU hCG at magnification × 2.5 and × 10, respectively. Antral follicles of size classes 1 to 5 are present. The highest magnification shows a healthy follicle of size class 4.

E and F Sections of ovaries after treatment with 8 IU recFSH and 2 IU hCG at magnification × 2.5 and × 10, respectively. Atretic antral follicles with dispersion of cumulus cells and a thin granulosa cell layer are apparent. The highest magnification shows a typical example of a size class 5 follicle without resumption of meiosis

Table 3 Effect of recFSH alone, recFSH supplemented with hCG and hCG alone in immature hypophysectomized rats treated twice daily for 4 days

Total dose (IU)			Ovarian weight	Uterine weight
recFSH	hCG	N^a	(mg)	(mg)
8	0	4	18.3 ± 2.8	19.5 ± 1.0
8	0.2	3	43.2 ± 9.3	106.3 ± 5.2*
8	0.5	4	32.1 ± 2.7	114.3 ± 5.3*
8	2	3	59.2 ± 7.4*	118.8 ± 5.6*
8	5	5	75.4 ± 5.8*	123.7 ± 3.2*
0	5	3	8.1 ± 1.0	16.0 ± 0.3

^{a}N represents the number of animals per treatment group.
*Significantly ($p < 0.05$) increased in comparison to treatment with 8 IU FSH only.

RecFSH with hCG

To evaluate the additional effect of LH activity, animals were treated with 8 IU recFSH supplemented with 0, 0.2, 0.5, 2, or 5 IU hCG. Controls were treated with 5 IU hCG only. Effects on ovarian and uterine weight are presented in Table 3.

Addition of hCG augmented ovarian weight significantly ($p < 0.05$) in a dose-dependent fashion, from 18.3 ± 2.8 mg in animals treated with 8 IU recFSH alone up to 75.4 ± 5.8 mg in those receiving the highest dose of hCG (5 IU). In contrast, even the lowest dose of hCG caused a maximal increase ($p < 0.05$) in uterine weight, from 19.5 ± 1.0 mg after treatment with 8 IU recFSH alone to 106.3 ± 5.2 mg after treatment with 8 IU recFSH and 0.2 IU hCG. Ovarian and uterine weights of animals treated with 5 IU hCG alone were similar to those of vehicle-treated animals.

The total number of healthy and atretic antral follicles and their distribution over the various size classes are depicted in Table 4 and Figure 2, respectively. Typical histological illustrations of ovarian sections are presented in Figure 4. In contrast to the effect on ovarian weight, the total number of antral follicles was further increased ($p < 0.05$) by only the highest dose of hCG, i.e., from 65 ± 8 per ovary after treatment with 8 IU recFSH alone to 105 ± 11 per ovary after treatment with 8 IU recFSH plus 5 IU hCG (Table 4). After treatment with 5 IU hCG alone, no antral follicles larger than 275 μm were present. In intact rats of the same age (30 days), the number of antral follicles was 42 ± 4 per ovary (Table 4), which is fourfold higher than in hypox vehicle-treated rats and about twofold lower than in hypox rats treated with at least

Table 4 Effect of recFSH supplemented with hCG on the number of healthy and atretic follicles in immature hypophysectomized rats

Treatment total dose (IU)			Total number of follicles (275μm)	Number of atretic follicles			Percentage of atretic follicles (>275μm)
recFSH	hCG	N^a		Early atretic[b]	Late atretic[c]	Other[d]	
8	0	4	65 ± 8	29 ± 5	9 ± 3	—	58 ± 2
8	0.2	3	89 ± 15	19 ± 11	—	—	20 ± 8
8	0.5	3	54 ± 14	2 ± 1	—	—	2 ± 8
8	2	3	67 ± 12	1 ± 1	4 ± 4	18 ± 6	31 ± 9
8	5	5	105 ± 11*	—	4 ± 2	25 ± 8	33 ± 4
0	5	5	—	—	—	—	—
intact	(day 30)	6	42 ± 4	6 ± 1	10 ± 2	—	39 ± 3

[a] N represents the number of animals per treatment group.
[b] Early atretic: stage 1a and 1b.
[c] Late atretic: stage 2a and 2b.
[d] Other: follicles with loosely arranged granulosa cells.
*Significantly ($p < 0.05$) increased in comparison to treatment with 8 IU FSH only.

10 IU recFSH alone (Table 2). In contrast to these latter rats, intact animals had only a few class 4 and no class 5 follicles.

In comparison to follicles in animals treated with 8 IU recFSH only, addition of as little as 0.2 IU hCG caused a pronounced shift from small (class 1 and 2) to large (class 4 and 5) antral follicles (Figure 2). Higher doses of hCG provided comparable size distributions.

In animals treated with 8 IU recFSH only, the incidence of atresia was 58% vs. 39% in intact animals (Table 4; Figure 4, A and B). This was due to a higher incidence of early atretic follicles (29 vs. 6). Supplementation with the lowest hCG doses, i.e., 0.2 and 0.5 IU, largely diminished the incidence of atresia to 20% and 2%, respectively (Table 4; Figure 4, C and D). Addition of 2 and 5 IU hCG induced class 4 and 5 follicles with a thin granulosa cell layer and loosely arranged granulosa cells (Figure 4, E and F), as did treatment with 40 IU recFSH only, resulting in 31% and 33% atretic follicles, respectively (Table 4).

DISCUSSION

The very first experiments in immature hypox rats, showing the synergistic effect of FSH and LH, date from the 1940s [10,11]. Thereafter, many comparable experiments were published (reviewed in [12]), sometimes with conflicting results due to the testing of FSH preparations with varying degrees of residual LH activity. Through the expression of FSH in mammalian host cells, pure human FSH devoid of LH has become available and allows definite elucidation of the specific action of FSH during follicular growth and steroidogenesis.

The current study in immature, hypox rats demonstrates that recFSH, in the complete absence of LH, increases the number of antral follicles and diminishes the incidence of atresia in these follicles. The effect on atresia was most apparent in the smallest follicle size class, indicating that FSH induces multiple follicular development by preventing small antral follicles from undergoing atresia. Furthermore, recFSH alone induced the growth of follicles to preovulatory stages, and subsequent administration of hCG resulted in ovulation of healthy follicles only, since large follicles with loosely arranged granulosa cells were still present after the induction of ovulation.

The above-described growth of ovulatory follicles confirms previous findings in hypox rodents treated with human FSH produced by recombinant DNA technology [13,14]. In the study by Galway et al. [14] with immature hypox rats, recFSH treatment without subsequent hCG administration could also induce ovulation. In these animals, however, a diethylstilbestrol capsule was implanted to prevent atresia after the withdrawal of gonadotropins. In our immature hypox rats, circulating E_2 remained at baseline. Although intraovarian E_2 increased in a recFSH dose-dependent manner, these levels were relatively low and were clearly suppressed due to the lack of LH activity since the highest dose of recFSH caused concentrations of E_2 comparable to those measurable in ovaries of intact immature animals, whereas the number of antral follicles was twice as high and these follicles were mainly of large size classes. Neither in hypox nor in intact animals was ovarian E_2 production sufficient to increase its concentration in the circulation.

In the current hypox model, ovarian androstenedione was undetectable, indicating that any available androgen substrate was immediately converted to estrogens. Production of androgens by ovarian theca interstitial cells might have occurred because of factors other than LH. For instance, in vitro studies on the control of androgen synthesis by thecal cells from rat and human ovaries have suggested that granulosa cell-derived inhibin enhances androgen production [15,16]. Furthermore, ovarian androgen biosynthesis is known to be promoted by insulin-like growth factor-1 of granulosa cell origin [17], which is also capable of augmenting FSH-induced estrogen biosynthesis [18].

Interestingly, uterine weight increased during recFSH treatment while plasma E_2 remained low at baseline, indicating that uterine weight is a more sensitive parameter for ovarian E_2 production than levels of serum E_2. So far, reports on uterine weight after recFSH treatment have been contradictory. After two days of recFSH treatment (total dose, 72 IU/hypox rat), Whitelaw and coworkers [19] found that uterine weights were not different from those of controls. However, in our study, treatment for four days with at least 10 IU recFSH per animal significantly increased uterine weight and caused endometrial proliferative growth. Increases of uterine weight have also been reported in adult hypox mice after recFSH treatment [13]. Previous measurements of intrauterine E_2 showed that recFSH-induced increases in uterine and ovarian E_2 are comparable [20], suggesting that estrogens produced by the ovaries bind to a uterine protein to cause local accumulation.

Supplementation of recFSH with hCG augmented ovarian weight, but except in the case of the highest hCG dose (5 IU), no further increases in the total number of follicles were observed. However, addition of only 0.2 to 0.5 IU hCG (doses sufficient to cause considerable increases in circulating E_2 and to augment ovarian aromatase activity [5]) caused a large shift of small follicles to preovulatory follicles. Also, addition of 0.5 IU hCG caused a large reduction in atresia in the various follicle size classes. Together these findings demonstrate that the number and quality of follicles are strongly determined by the FSH/LH ratio of gonadotropins used to induce superovulation. For administering hCG in the hypox rat, a ratio of 16:1 (8 IU FSH:0.5 IU hCG) might be most favorable, although additional dose-finding and time-course experiments would be required to substantiate these data.

The present study also demonstrated that doses of FSH and hCG that are too high are detrimental for normal follicular development. After treatment with 40 IU (200 IU/ kg/day) of recFSH alone or after treatment with 8 IU recFSH and 2 to 5 IU hCG, 20 to 25% of antral follicles had lost their compact structure with respect to the granulosa cell layer and showed loosely arranged cumulus cells, suggesting secretion of an excess of follicular fluid. Most likely, these follicles represent an abnormal stage of atresia as indicated by the results after prolonged treatment with recFSH. The follicles with a thin layer of granulosa cells present after combined treatment with 8 IU recFSH and 2 or 5 IU hCG probably develop to cystic follicles as described by Bogovich [21], who treated immature hypox rats with ovine FSH and hCG for 2 weeks. Obviously these findings are of interest for understanding ovarian pathophysiological processes, but the doses required to induce these processes were extremely high – much higher than those applied to induce superovulation in animals or humans.

In summary, recFSH alone is able to induce follicle growth up to the preovulatory stage, mainly by preventing small antral follicles from undergoing atresia; but small amounts of LH amity, either exogenous or endogenous, are beneficial during recFSH-induced multiple follicular growth in that the number of healthy follicles is enlarged. In the complete absence of LH activity, recFSH increases uterine weight by stimulating proliferate growth of the endometrium.

ACKNOWLEDGEMENTS

The authors wish to express their gratitude to Mr. C. Strijbos and co-workers, Mrs E. van Leeuwen, Mr. B Karels, and Mr. A van Ravestein for their skilful technical assistance and to E. de Rijk, Ph.D., for the quantitation of the uterine epithelium. The critical review of this manuscript by Dr H. Kloosterboer is highly appreciated.

REFERENCES

1. Chappel SC, Howles C. Reevaluation of the roles of luteinizing hormone and follicle-stimulating hormone in the ovulatory process. Hum Reprod 1991; 6:1206–1212.
2. Baird DT. A model for follicular selection and ovulation: lessons from superovulation. J Steroid Biochem 1987; 27:15–23.
3. Glasier AF, Baird DT, Hillier SG. FSH and the control of follicular growth. J Steroid Biochem 1989; 32:167–170.
4. Hsueh AJW, Adashi EY, Jones PBC, Welsh TH. Hormonal regulation of the differentiation of cultured granulosa cells. Endocr Rev 1984; 5:76–127.
5. Mannaerts B, De Leeuw R, Geelen J, Van Ravenstein A, Van Wezenbeek P, Schuurs A, Kloosterboer H. Comparative in vitro and in vivo studies on the biological properties of recombinant human follicle stimulating hormone. Endocrinology 1991; 129:2623-2630.
6. Shoham Z, Balen A, Patel A, Jacobs H. Results of ovulation induction using human menopausal gonadotropins or purified follicle-stimulating hormone in hypogonadotropic hypogonadism patients. Fertil Steril 1991; 56:1048–1053.
7. Schoot BC, Coelingh Bennink HJ, Mannaerts BM, Lamberts SW, Bouchard P, Fauser BC. Human recombinant follicle-stimulating hormone induces growth of preovulatory follicles without concomitant increase in androgen and estrogen biosynthesis in a woman with isolated gonadotropin deficiency. J Clin Endocrinol Metab 1992; 74:1471–1473.
8. Shoham Z, Mannaerts B, Insler V, Coelingh Bennink H. Induction of follicular growth using recombinant human follicle-stimulating hormone in two volunteer women with hypogonadotropic hypogonadism. Fertil Steril 1993; 59:738–742.
9. Osman P. Rate and course of atresia during follicular development in the adult cyclic rat. J Reprod Fertil 1985; 73:261–270.
10. Fevold HL. Synergism of follicle stimulating and luteinizing hormone in producing estrogen secretion. Endocrinology 1941; 28:33–36.

11. Greep RO, VanDyke HB, Chow BF. Gonadotropins of the swine pituitary 1. Various biological effects of purified thylakentrin (FSH) and pure metakentrin (ICSH). Endocrinology 1942; 30 635–649.
12. Richards JS. Maturation of ovarian follicles: actions and interactions of pituitary and ovarian hormones on follicular cell differentiations. Physiol Rev 1980, 60:51–89.
13. Wang X, Greenwald GS. Human chorionic gonadotropin or human recombinant follicle-stimulating hormone (FSH)-induced ovulation and subsequent fertilization and early embryo development in hypophysectomized FSH-primed mice. Endocrinology 1993; 132:2009–2016.
14. Galway AB, Lapolt PS, Tsafriri A, Dargan CM, Boime I, Hsueh AJW. Recombinant follicle-stimulating hormone induces ovulation and tissue plasminogen activator expression in hypophysectomized rats. Endocrinology 1990,127:3023–3028.
15. Hsueh AJW, Dahl KD, Vaughan J, Tucker E, Rivier J, Bardin CW, Vale W. Heterodimers and homodimers of inhibin subunits have different paracrine action in the modulation of luteinizing hormone-stimulated androgen biosynthesis. Proc Natl Acad Sci USA 1987; 84:5082–5086.
16. Hillier SG, Yong EL, Illingworth PJ, Baird DT, Schwall RH, Mason AJ. Effect of recombinant inhibin on androgen synthesis in cultured human thecal cells. Mol Cell Endocrinol 1991; 75:R1–R6.
17. Hernandez ER, Roberts CT Jr, Hurwitz A, LeRoith D, Adashi EY. Somatomedin C/insulin-like growth factor I as an enhancer of androgen biosynthesis by cultured rat ovarian cells. Endocrinology 1988; 122:1603–1612.
18. Adashi EY, Resnick CE, Hurwitz A, Ricciarellie E, Hernandez ER, Roberts CT, Leroith D, Rosenfeld R. The intraovarian IGF system. Growth Regul 1992; 2:10–19.
19. Whitelaw PF, Smyth CD, Howles CM, Hillier SG. Cell-specific expression of aromatase and LH receptor mRNAs in rat ovary. J Mol Endocrinol 1993; 9:309–312.
20. De Leeuw R, Van Ravestein A, Geelen J, Mannaerts B, Kloosterboer H. Pharmacodynamics of recombinant FSH in immature, hypophysectomized female rats. In: The 8th annual meeting of the ESHRE; 1992; The Hague. Abstract 107.
21. Bogovich K. Follicle-stimulating hormone plays a role in the induction of ovarian follicular cysts in hypophysectomized rats. Biol Reprod 1992; 47:149–161.

Received November 16, 1993; accepted March 16, 1994

Correspondence: Bernadette Mannaerts, Medical R&D Unit, NV Organon, PO Box 20, 5340 BH Oss, The Netherlands. FAX 4120-62617/62555

Section II

Clinical aspects

5

First established pregnancy and birth after ovarian stimulation with recombinant human follicle stimulating hormone (Org 32489)

P. Devroey[*], B.M.J.L. Mannaerts[†], J. Smitz[*], H.J.T. Coelingh Bennink[†] and A. Van Steirteghem[*]

[*]Center for Reproductive Medicine, Free University of Brussels, Laarbeeklaan 101, 1090 Brussels, Belgium and [†]Medical R & D Unit, NV Organon, PO Box 20, 5340 BH Oss, The Netherlands

ABSTRACT

This case report describes the first established pregnancy and birth after ovarian stimulation with Org 32489, pure recombinant human follicle stimulating hormone (recFSH, NV Organon). A patient with tubal infertility participated in an open efficacy study of recFSH evaluating the efficacy of combined gonadotrophin-releasing hormone (GnRH)-agonist/recFSH treatment in women undergoing in-vitro fertilization (IVF) and embryo transfer. Ovarian stimulation was induced by recFSH in association with buserelin (Suprecur®, $4 \times 150\,\mu g$/day) using a short protocol. After 9 days of recFSH treatment (75 IU/day), six pre-ovulatory follicles (≥ 15 mm) were observed and 10 000 IU human chorionic gonadotrophin were administered. Nine mature oocytes were retrieved by oocyte puncture and after IVF, three embryos were replaced in the uterus. A viable singleton intra-uterine pregnancy was revealed at a gestational age of 7 weeks. The pregnancy progressed normally and ended with a vaginal delivery at a gestational age of 39.5 weeks. A healthy girl was born and paediatric examination did not demonstrate any abnormality.

This case report was first published in *Human Reproduction*, **8** (6), 863–865 (1993). Copyright 1993 Oxford University Press, reproduced with permission

CASE REPORT

A 29-year-old patient and her 31-year-old husband had been infertile since 1984. In 1990 an ectopic pregnancy with tubal rupture occurred and a subsequent salpingectomy by laparotomy was done elsewhere. During laparoscopic examination in 1991, the remaining Fallopian tube was found to be severely damaged, but ovarian function was normal as judged by serial measurements of serum follicle stimulating hormone (FSH), luteinizing hormone (LH), oestradiol and progesterone. Hysteroscopy, semen analysis and karyotype analysis of both partners showed no abnormalities. Subsequently, the couple gave informed consent to participate in an open study with recombinant FSH (recFSH) (Org 32489) evaluating the efficacy of combined gonadotrophin-releasing hormone (GnRH)-agonist/recFSH therapy in women undergoing in-vitro fertilization (IVF) and embryo transfer.

Women of infertile couples participating in this study were allocated to different treatment groups including treatment with recFSH only (group 1) and treatment with recFSH in conjunction with pituitary desensitization using buserelin intranasal spray (Suprecur® $4\times150\,\mu g$/day, in a short protocol (group 2) or a long protocal (group 3), or using tryptorelin (Decapeptyl®) in a long protocol giving a single dose of 3.75 mg i.m. (group 4) or daily s.c. injections of 200 μg (group 5). The patient reported here was allocated to group 2. The study was approved by the Belgian Health Authorities and the Ethics Committee of the Brussels Free University Hospital, and the results will be reported separately.

In the case reported here, recFSH was administered i.m. in a daily dose of 75 IU (calibrated as urinary FSH/human menopausal gonadotrophin (HMG) preparations with the Steelman and Pohley bioassay) from menstrual cycle days 3–11. Buserelin intake was started 1 day before the first FSH injection. Follicular growth and serum FSH, LH, progesterone, oestradiol and inhibin were monitored on several treatment days and are presented in Table 1. Serum LH gradually declined from 3.8 IU/l on cycle day 1 to 0.9 IU/l on cycle day 11 whereas progesterone remained low. After several treatment days, serum FSH concentrations (3–5 IU/l) were comparable to that measured on cycle day 1. In contrast, a 2-fold increase of serum inhibin was noted and serum oestradiol concentration increased rapidly from 36 pg/ml on cycle day 1 up to 2640 pg/ml on cycle day 12 when six pre-ovulatory follicles (diameter 15–23 mm) were observed by vaginal ultrasonography. Subsequently, resumption of meiosis was induced by human chorionic gonadotrophin (HCG; 10 000 IU Pregnyl®, NV Organon, Oss, The Netherlands) and 36 h later nine mature oocytes (type 1.0 according to the criteria of Staessen et al., 1989) were retrieved by ultrasonographically

Table 1 Follicular growth and hormone concentrations during recombinant follicle stimulating hormone (recFSH) treatment

Cycle day	No. of follicles according to size (mm)			Oestradiol (pg/ml)	Inhibin (IU/l)	FSH (IU/l)	LH (IU/l)	Progesterone (µg/l)
	12–14	15–16	≥17					
1	0	0	0	36	5.2	5	3.8	0.2
6	2	0	0	246	5.2	3	2.6	<0.1
8				592	6.4	5	0.5	<0.1
9	1	5	1	760	6.6	4	0.9	<0.1
10				1144	7.9	3	0.8	<0.1
11				1545	10.6	4	0.9	0.1
12	0	2	4	2640	—	4	1.8	0.3

LH = luteinizing hormone; FSH = follicle stimulating hormone.

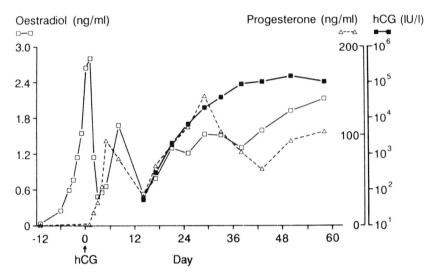

Figure 1 Serum oestradiol levels during recombinant follicle stimulating hormone (recFSH) treatment before the day of human chorionic gonadotrophin (HCG) administration (day 0) and serum oestradiol, progesterone and HCG levels up to 60 days after embryo transfer. A turning-point of oestradiol and progesterone production is obvious 2 weeks after HCG injection

guided vaginal methods. In total four oocytes were fertilized and three 4-cell embryos were transferred into the uterus and one 4-cell embryo was cryopreserved.

The luteal phase was supported by means of vaginally administered micronized natural progesterone (600 mg/day, Utrogestan®, Piette, Belgium). Serum progesterone, oestradiol and HCG concentrations were measured at regular intervals during the first 2 months after HCG administration and are depicted in Figure 1. During the first week after HCG, an initial rise of serum oestradiol and progesterone was apparent. Thereafter, these steroids started to decline, but 1 week later a secondary rise of progesterone and oestradiol was noted due to rapidly increasing HCG levels, indicating that the subject was pregnant. A viable singleton intra-uterine pregnancy was observed by means of ultrasonography at a gestational age of 7 weeks (day 38 after HCG). No fetal abnormalities were revealed by ultrasound scans performed during the second and third trimester. The pregnancy progressed normally and ended with a vaginal delivery at a gestational age of 39.5 weeks. A healthy girl was born weighing 3170 g and having an Apgar score of 9/10 (1/5 min). Paediatric examination of the baby did not demonstrate any abnormality. Overall, the treatment was well tolerated and no adverse effects were noted.

DISCUSSION

In 1978, Steptoe and Edwards reported on the birth of Louise Brown, the first baby born following reimplantation of an in-vitro fertilized oocyte. In the next decade, assisted reproduction by means of ovarian stimulation with HMG and IVF/embryo transfer (ET) developed rapidly and the efficacy and safety of urinary gonadotrophins was unequivocally proven by the thousands of healthy babies born following this treatment. This year, we report on the first established pregnancy and subsequent birth after ovarian stimulation with a new biosynthetic FSH preparation (Devroey et al., 1992a,b).

The patient described received recFSH in association with buserelin in a short protocol. The latter, known to cause an initial rise of endogenous FSH and LH, is likely to be responsible for the very low dose of recFSH (total dose 675 IU; 75 IU/day) required to induce ovarian stimulation. Interestingly after several treatment days, circulating FSH remained constant and was comparable to that measured on cycle day 1, whereas serum oestradiol increased rapidly and simultaneous follicular growth was noted.

The application of recFSH devoid of (intrinsic) LH activity (Mannaerts et al., 1991) may be indicated for ovulation induction or ovarian stimulation. Currently, treatment for these indications frequently utilizes a GnRH agonist, to suppress endogenous levels of LH and/or premature LH surges. In most conditions, enough endogenous LH is available to support FSH-induced folliculogenesis. Clinical research, however, should also elucidate whether in gonadotrophin-deficient women (Schoot et al., 1992) or in patients with severe pituitary suppression the amount of remaining endogenous LH is sufficient to support FSH-induced steroidogenesis. It is expected that this IVF study, evaluating the efficacy of various combined GnRH/recFSH regimens may provide further insight into the requirements of LH during ovulation induction. Preliminary evaluation of the data has revealed that successful ovulation induction and pregnancies are established regardless of the GnRH regimen applied but that the remaining endogenous LH determines the total amount of recFSH required for successful ovulation. These data suggest that the remaining LH activity influences the initial ovarian responsiveness rather than the actual treatment outcome. Further clinical research is required to confirm these preliminary findings and to assess the long-term safety and efficacy of recFSH in comparison to urinary gonadotrophins, with special emphasis on the avoidance of multiple pregnancy and hyperstimulation.

ACKNOWLEDGEMENTS

The authors gratefully acknowledge the skilful assistance of study co-ordinator Ms A. de Brabanter and study monitor Mr G. Lathouwers.

REFERENCES

Devroey, P., Van Steirteghem, A., Mannaerts, B. and Coelingh Bennink, H. (1992a) Successful in-vitro fertilization and embryo transfer after treatment with recombinant human FSH. *Lancet,* **339**, 1170–1171.

Devroey, P., Van Steirteghem, A., Mannaerts, B. and Coelingh Bennink, H. (1992b) First singleton term birth after ovarian superovulation with recombinant human follicle stimulating hormone (Org 32489). *Lancet,* **340**, 1108.

Mannaerts, B., De Leeuw, R., Geelen, J., Van Ravenstein, A., Van Wezenbeek, P., Schuurs, A. and Kloosterboer, L. (1991) Comparative in vitro and in vivo studies on the biological properties of recombinant human follicle stimulating hormone. *Endocrinology,* **129**, 2623–2630.

Schoot, B.C., Coelingh Bennink, H.J., Mannaerts, B.M., Lamberts, S.W., Bouchard, P. and Fauser, B.C. (1992) Human recombinant follicle-stimulating hormone induces growth of preovulatory follicles without concomitant increase in androgen and estrogen biosynthesis in a woman with isolated gonadotrophin deficiency. *J. Clin. Endocrinol. Metab.,* **74**, 1471–1473.

Staessen, C., Camus, M., Khan, I., Smitz, J., Van Waesberghe, L., Wisanto, A., Devroey, P. and Van Steirteghem, A.C. (1989) An 18-month survey of infertility treatment by in vitro fertilization, gamete and zygote intrafallopian transfer, and replacement of frozen-thawed embryos. *J. In Vitro Fertil. Embryo Transfer,* **6**, 22–29.

Steptoe, P.C. and Edwards, R.G. (1978) Birth after the reimplantation of a human embryo. *Lancet,* **ii**, 366.

Received October 28, 1992; accepted February 18, 1993

Correspondence: P. Devroey, Center for Reproductive Medicine, Free University of Brussels, Laarbeeklaan 101, 1090 Brussels, Belgium

6

Human recombinant follicle-stimulating hormone induces growth of preovulatory follicles without concomitant increase in androgen and estrogen biosynthesis in a woman with isolated gonadotropin deficiency

*D.C. Schoot, H.J.T. Coelingh Bennink,
B.M.J.L. Mannaerts, S.W.J. Lamberts,
P. Bouchard and B.C.J.M. Fauser*

Section of Reproductive Endocrinology and Infertility, Department of Obstetrics and Gynecology; Department of Medicine, Dijkzigt University Hospital, Rotterdam; Scientific Development Group, NV Organon, Oss, The Netherlands; and Service d'Endocrinologie et des Maladies de la Reproduction, Hôpital Bicêtre, Paris, France

ABSTRACT

To evaluate the importance of luteinizing hormone (LH) for normal estrogen production and subsequent development of ovarian follicles, a woman with isolated gonadotropin deficiency (LH; 0.37 IU/L, FSH 1.2 IU/L) was monitored during recombinant human follicle-stimulating hormone (hFSHrec) administration with respect to ovarian follicular growth and steroid production. During the first week (75 IU/day hFSHrec im) a significant rise in serum FSH (4.9 IU/L) was observed in the absence of changes in serum estradiol (E2) concentrations (36–76 pmol/L). During the following five days 150 IU/day hFSHrec was administered resulting in a further increase of serum FSH levels (maximum 8.5 IU/L). Development of multiple follicles – maximum diameter 22 mm as observed by transvaginal sonography – emerged together with a minor rise in E2 levels (from 76 to 236 pmol/L) and with a minimal increase in endometrial thickness (below 6 mm). Six days following the *last injection of hFSHrec, aspiration of 3 follicles (13, 15 and 18 mm) was performed and low intrafollicular androstenedione (AD) (<675 nmol/L) and E2 (<9400 pmol/L) concentrations as compared to normal follicles were found. These first data on hFSHrec administration in the human suggest that; a) FSH alone can induce growth of preovulatory follicles, b) follicle growth does occur in the presence of subnormal E2 levels, c) LH is needed for adequate AD biosynthesis as substrate for aromatase activity. This indicates that growth and steroidogenic granulosa cell activity may be differently regulated.*

INTRODUCTION

Chinese hamster ovary (CHO) cells transfected with human follicle-stimulating hormone (FSH) subunit genes are capable of secreting the intact FSH dimer (1). Moreover, the biological activity of human recombinant FSH (hFSHrec) was ascertained using rat granulosa cell cultures and intact immature rats (2,3). Commercially available preparations of purified urinary gonadotropins may have varying molecular composition (4), and all available preparations contain varying degrees of luteinizing hormone (LH). Although hFSHrec also consists of a mixture of FSH isohormones, bioactivity appears identical to pituitary FSH, without LH bioactivity (3).

The hypothesis of gonadotropin synergism, introduced almost half a century ago (5) emphasized the importance of an interplay between LH and FSH for normal estrogen production and follicular development. This concept was supported by observations in infantile mice after injection of pure urinary FSH (6). The observed increase in ovarian weight in combination with absent uterine growth, suggested that FSH alone is incapable of initiating estrogen production but still leads to follicular development. Moreover, the administration of purified FSH in hypogonadotropic women resulted in normal follicular development and low serum estrogen levels (7). An ongoing study using hFSHrec in hypogonadotropic subjects to assess safety and pharmacokinetical characteristics of the drug, provided an unique opportunity to explore whether LH exposure is essential for the induction of adequate estrogen production and subsequent follicle growth.

PATIENT AND METHODS

A healthy female (age; 39 yrs, weight; 53 kg) suffering from primary amenorrhea due to isolated congenital gonadotropin deficiency, volunteered to enter an open phase I clinical trial with hFSHrec to assess its tolerance, safety, pharmacokinetic and pharmacodynamic properties. Serum levels were 0.37 IU/L for LH and 1.2 IU/L for FSH. The study was approved by the Ethics Review Committee of the Erasmus University/Dijkzigt Hospital and informed consent was obtained. Wish for procreation was absent. Three successful gonadotropin induced pregnancies (one twin pregnancy) had been established previously. Physical examination and routine urine/serum examinations were normal. Autoimmunity was excluded by anti-nuclear (ANA) and specific anti-FSH (anti-Org 32489) antibody assays.

She refrained from estrogen replacement therapy 10 days prior to this study.

hFSHrec (Org 32489; NV Organon, Oss, The Netherlands) was administered in a daily dose of 75 IU (standardized according to the Steelman/Pohley in vivo FSH bioassay (3)) im for 7 days, followed by 150 IU/day during week 2. Medication was discontinued according to protocol criteria, because one ovarian follicle was found to exceed a diameter of 14 mm on day 13. On day 19, multiple follicles (n = 6; 12–18 mm) were observed. After informed consent was obtained 3 follicles (13, 15, and 18 mm diameter) were punctured (no oocytes were obtained; fluid was stored separately) and 10,000 IU human chorionic gonadotropin (hCG) (Pregnyl; NV Organon) was administered im.

Blood withdrawal and pelvic sonography on alternate days was continued for 3 weeks following the last hFSHrec injection. Transvaginal sonography, using a 5 mHz transducer (Model 1550; Philips Medical Systems, Eindhoven, The Netherlands), was performed as published previously (8). Endometrial thickness was measured between the two parallel (opposite) hyperechogenic myometrium–endometrium interfaces. The largest distance, measured in the sagittal plane, representing two layers of endometrium, was recorded. For reference values, fluid was obtained from 118 individual non-dominant follicles (3–9 mm diameter) between cycle day 2–12 in 16 regularly cycling women (control) (9), and from 7 dominant follicles (13–24 mm diameter), between cycle day 10 and 12, from 7 regularly cycling women. Serum and follicular fluid was centrifuged and stored at –20°C. Immunoreactive LH and FSH serum levels were assessed in one assay using a immunoradiometric assay (IRMA) kit (Delfia, Pharmacia, Woerden, The Netherlands). Data are expressed in terms of MRC 78/549 for FSH and MRC 80/552 for LH. Intra-assay coefficients of variation were less than 4.8% for FSH and less than 4.7% for LH. Estradiol (E2) levels in serum and follicular fluid were estimated by radioimmunoassay (RIA) (Diagnostics Products Corp. Los Angeles, CA) (9, 10). Progesterone (P) was measured in serum by RIA using an antibody against 11α-hydroxyprogesterone-hemisuccinate bovine serum albumin complex. Serum and follicular androstenedione (AD) levels were measured using the antiserum described by Frölich and coworkers (11), after extraction with diethyl ether. Intra-assay coefficients of variation were less than 5% for E2, and less than 7% for AD. The anti-FSH antibody assay used labelled Org 32489 as a ligand and mouse antibodies raised against Org 32489 as a reference (detection limit: 0.5 pmol/L). ANA was measured using immunofluorescence technique in a Hep-2 cell line (Bio-Lab, Amersfoort, The Netherlands).

RESULTS

Baseline hormonal parameters showed confirmation of the hypogonadotropic hypogonadal state (FSH; 1.2 IU/L, LH; 0.37 IU/L, E2; 63 pmol/L). Thyroid-stimulating hormone, prolactin and cortisol levels were within normal limits (data not shown). Sonography before hFSHrec administration, showed follicles at a size below 4 mm in each ovary (Figure 1). Follicular development started, after the daily dosage was increased from 1 to 2 ampules hFSHrec on day 7. Following the last hFSHrec injection (day 12), multiple ovarian follicles increased in size (maximum 22 mm). After puncture, two follicles of more than 14 mm remained. Following hCG injection, follicles decreased gradually in size. Endometrial thickness increased by 2 mm during the treatment period (from 4 to 6 mm) (Figure 1).

A rise in serum FSH levels was observed during hFSHrec administration with a maximum concentration of 8.5 IU/L (Figure 1), followed by a decrease up to 1.3 IU/L on the day of hCG administration. Serum LH concentrations varied between 0.09 and 0.38 IU/L before hCG administration, and no systemic changes did occur. Serum E2 levels showed a gradual increase to a maximum of 236 pmol/L on day 15 (day of maximum follicular size) (Figure 2a). Serum P showed no elevation following hCG administration (data not shown).

Fluid obtained from the largest follicle (18 mm) revealed an E2 concentration of 9400 pmol/L, and AD was 675 nmol/L. The remaining two follicles (15 and 13 mm) showed E2 and AD concentrations of 3800 pmol/L, 160 nmol/L and 3100 pmol/L, 115 nmol/L respectively (Figure 2b). Concentrations of both FSH and LH were below detection limits in follicular fluid (data not shown). In normal small (3–9 mm) follicles (n = 118) the median E2 level was 91 (range 1.5–7000) × 1000 pmol/L, and AD levels 3160 (330–9580) nmol/L. In normal large (13–24 mm) follicles (n = 7) E2 levels were 14563 (10657–20446) ×1000 pmol/L, and AD levels 3000 (620–5480) nmol/L.

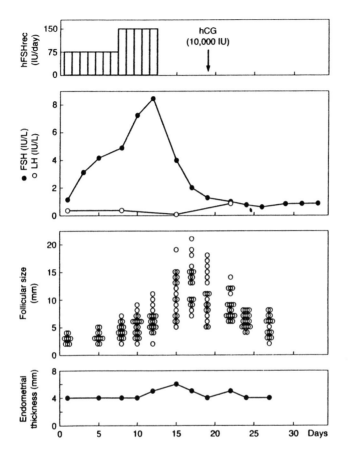

Figure 1 hFSHrec and hCG dose regimens administered to a patient with isolated gonadotropin deficiency, serum FSH (IU/L) and LH (IU/L) levels in the upper two panels. Diameters (mm) of separate follicles as determined by vaginal sonography for both ovaries, and sonographic estimation of endometrial thickness (mm) in the lower two panels

DISCUSSION

This study represents the first data on hFSHrec administration in the human. No adverse effects and no anti-hFSHrec antibody formation was observed. Development of follicles occurred following administration of increasing amounts of hFSHrec, similar to what is observed following exogenous gonadotropins used for induction of ovulation. Following the last injection of hFSHrec follicular development continued towards pre-ovulatory sizes whereas FSH concentrations decreased, in keeping with previous observations (12) suggesting that

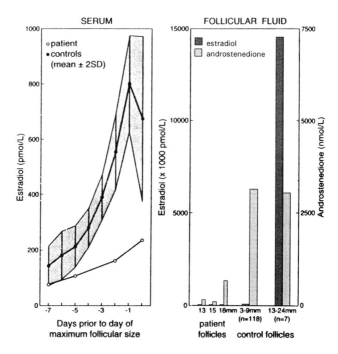

Figure 2a Serum estradiol (pmol/L) concentrations of a patient with isolated gonadotropin deficiency following hFSHrec administration prior to the day where ovarian follicles reach their maximum size (day 17). As a reference, daily serum estradiol levels (mean ± 2SD) are shown in seven normally cycling women up to the day of LH peak (see also ref. 11). **Figure 2b** Estradiol (E2)(pmol/L) and androstenedione (AD)(nmol/L) follicular fluid concentrations in three separate follicles (13, 15, 18 mm diameter) in a patient with isolated gonadotropin deficiency after hFSHrec administration. Median E2 and AD concentrations in small (3–9 mm) follicles (n = 118), and large (13–24 mm) follicles (n = 7)

growth of dominant follicles may be less dependent on circulating FSH concentrations.

Based on previous studies in the rat it is generally believed that estrogens are essential for normal follicular development. Recent clinical observations suggest that this concept may need to be revised for the human (13). For instance, ovarian follicular development could be induced in a woman with inadequate estrogen and androgen biosynthesis due to 17α-hydroxylase deficiency (14). In addition, it appears that normal follicular growth can be induced using purified urinary FSH preparations (7). In the present study, in sharp contrast to normal follicular development, E2 levels remained low. Observed levels around day 15 are similar to early follicular phase E2 concentrations in normal cycles (12) (Figure 2a). The minor increase in endometrial thickness is also in favour of minimal estrogen bioactivity. E2 and AD concentrations in 3 aspirated large follicles appear to be extremely low, as compared to concentrations in small and large follicles in controls (Figure 2b). This indicates that ovarian follicles are incapable of producing sufficient amounts of AD in the presence of minute amounts of LH (below 0.38 IU/L). The subsequent inability of normal estrogen production within follicles is in keeping with the two cell two gonadotropin hypothesis, indicating that FSH induced granulosa cell aromatase activity can only lead to augmented E2 production if a sufficient amount of the aromatase substrate AD is available. This underlines the concept of a LH threshold for sufficient estrogen production. It was surprising indeed, that the mitogenic activity induced by FSH (i.e. proliferation of granulosa cells (15) did take place in a local environment with extremely low estrogen concentrations. This observation points to a differential regulation by FSH of steroidogenic and mitogenic granulosa cell activity. Direct effects of local estrogens on oocyte development are unknown.

Various reasons could explain the absence of a rise in serum P level following the injection of hCG. It may be hypothesized, based on in vitro observations (16), that physiological FSH levels in combination with low local E2 concentrations, as observed in the present subject, were insufficient for the induction of LH receptors, and that these follicles were therefore not responsive to hCG. The possibility that declining FSH serum levels caused a decrease in number of LH receptors (17) on the day of hCG administration cannot be ruled out. In addition, remaining follicles may have been too small for adequate hCG response.

In summary, data presented in this study indicate the significance of sufficient amounts of LH – next to FSH – for adequate E2 production by ovarian follicles and further suggest differential regulation of mitogenic and steroidogenic granulosa cell activity by FSH. Since FSH alone – in the absence of LH – can induce growth of preovulatory follicles, it seems questionable whether estrogen biosynthesis is mandatory for follicular development in the human. For induction of ovulation, however, sufficient estrogen concentrations seem important for production of cervical mucus and normal endometrial function.

ACKNOWLEDGEMENTS

The authors are grateful to the staff of the immunoassay laboratory (head; Dr F.H. de Jong) and the clinical research department ('Balans afdeling') for their assistance. Dr T.D. Pache is kindly acknowledged for collecting the follicular fluid samples.

REFERENCES

1. Keene JL, Matzuk MM, Otani T et al. Expression of biologically active human follitropin in chinese hamster ovary cells. J Biol Chem. 1989;246:4769–75.
2. Galway AB, Hsueh AJW, Keene JL, Yamoto M, Fauser BCJM, Biome I. In vitro and in vivo bioactivity of recombinant follicle-stimulating hormone and partially deglycosylated variants secreted by transfected eukaryotic cell lines. Endocrinology. 1990;127:93–9.
3. Mannaerts B, de Leeuw R, Geelen J, et al. Comparative in vitro and in vivo studies on the biological characteristics of recombinant human follicle stimulating hormone. Endocrinology. 1991;129:2623–30.
4. Harlin J, Kahn SA, Diczfaluzy E. Molecular composition of luteinizing hormone and follicle stimulating hormone in commercial gonadotropin preparations. Fertil Steril. 1986;46:1055–60.
5. Fevold HL. Synergism of follicle stimulating and luteinizing hormone in producing estrogen secretion. Endocrinology. 1941;28:33–6.
6. Eshkol A, Lunenfeld B. Purification and separation of follicle stimulating hormone (FSH) and luteinizing hormone from human menopausal gonadotropin; III. Effects of a biologically apparently pure FSH preparation on ovaries and uteri of intact immature mice. Acta Endocrinol (Copenh). 1967;54:91–5.
7. Couzinet B, Lestrat N, Brailly S, Forest M, Schaison G. Stimulation of ovarian follicular maturation with pure follicle stimulating hormone in women with gonadotropin deficiency. J Clin Endocrinol Metab. 1988;66:552–6.
8. Pache TD, Wladimiroff JW, de Jong FH, Hop WC, Fauser BCJM. Growth patterns of nondominant follicles during the normal menstrual cycles. Fertil Steril. 1990;54:638–42.
9. Pache TD, Hop WCJ, de Jong FH et al. Oestradiol, androstenedione and inhibin levels in individual follicles from normal and polycystic ovaries, and ovaries from androgen treated female to male transsexuals. Clin Endocrinol (Oxf). In Press.
10. Fauser BCJM, Pache TD, Lamberts SWJ, Hop WCJ, de Jong FH, Dahl KD. Serum bioactive and immunoreactive luteinizing hormone and follicle-stimulating hormone levels in women with cycle abnormalities, with or without polycystic ovarian disease. J Clin Endocrinol Metab. 1991;73:811–7.
11. Frölich M, Brand EC, van Hall EV. Serum levels of unconjugated aetiocholanolone, androstenedione, testosterone, dehydroepiandrosterone, aldosterone, progesterone, and oestrogens during the normal menstrual cycle. Acta Endocrinol (Copenh). 1976;81:548–62.

12. Schoot DC, Pache TD, Hop WC, de Jong FH, Fauser BCJM. Growth patterns of ovarian follicles during induction of ovulation with decreasing doses of human menopausal gonadotropin following presumed selection in polycystic ovary syndrome patients. Fertil Steril. In Press.
13. Chappel SC, Howles C. Reevaluation of the roles of luteinizing hormone and follicle stimulating hormone in the ovulatory process. Hum Reprod. 1991;9:1206–12.
14. Rabinovici J, Blankstein J, Goldman B, et al. In vitro fertilization and primary embryonic cleavage are possible in 17α-hydroxylase deficiency despite extremely low intrafollicular 17β-estradiol. J Clin Endocrinol Metab. 1991;68:693–7.
15. Rao MC, Rees Midgley A Jr, Richards JS. Hormonal regulation of ovarian cellular proliferation. Cell. 1978;14:71–8.
16. Kessel B, Liu YX, Jia XC, Hsueh AJW. Autocrine role of estrogens in the augmentation of luteinizing hormone receptor formation in cultured rat granulosa cells. Biol Reprod. 1985;32:1038–50.
17. Jia X, Hsueh AJW. Homologous regulation of hormone receptors: luteinizing hormone increases its own receptors in cultured rat granulosa cells. Endocrinology. 1984;115:2433–9.

Correspondence: Dr B.C.J.M. Fauser, Section of Reproductive Endocrinology and Infertility, Department of Obstetrics and Gynecology, Dijkzigt University Hospital, Dr. Molewaterplein 40, 3015 GD Rotterdam, The Netherlands

7

Single-dose pharmacokinetics and pharmocodynamics of recombinant human follicle-stimulating hormone (Org 32489) in gonadotropin-deficient volunteers

B.M.J.L. Mannaerts*, Z. Shoham[†], D. Schoot[‡], P. Bouchard[§],
J. Harlin[¶], B. Fauser[‡], H. Jacobs[†], F. Rombout* and H.J.T. Coelingh Bennink*

*Scientific Development Group, NV Organon, Oss, The Netherlands; [†]Cobbold Laboratories, Middlesex Hospital, London, UK; [‡]Department of Obstetrics and Gynecology, Dijkzigt University Hospital, Rotterdam, The Netherlands; [§]Service d'Endocrinologie et de Maladies de la Reproduction, Hôpital Bicêtre, France; [¶]Department of Obstetrics and Gynecology, Karolinska Hospital, Stockholm, Sweden

ABSTRACT

Objective: *To assess safety, pharmacokinetic, and pharmacodynamic properties of recombinant human follicle-stimulating hormone (FSH; Org 32489, NV Organon, Oss, The Netherlands) after a single intramuscular injection in the buttock.*
Design: *In a prospective study, safety variables, serum FSH, luteinizing hormone, inhibin, estradiol (females only), and testosterone (males only) were evaluated up to a maximum of 11 days after injection of 300 IU recombinant FSH.*
Setting: *Four specialist Reproductive Endocrinology and Infertility units.*
Volunteers: *Fifteen men and women exhibiting all pituitary gonadotropin deficiency.*
Results: *A single bolus of 300 IU recombinant FSH was well tolerated, and no drug-related adverse effects were noted. Comparison of before and after treatment safety variables, including serum antirecombinant*

This paper was first published in *Fertility and Sterility*, **59** (1), 108–114 (1993). Reproduced with permission of the publisher, the American Society for Reproductive Medicine (formerly The American Fertility Society)

FSH antibodies, showed no changes of clinical relevance. Analysis of serum FSH levels revealed comparable elimination half-lives of 44 ± 14 (mean ± SD) and 32 ± 12 hours in women and men volunteers, respectively. In contrast, peak FSH concentrations were significantly lower in women than in men volunteers (4.3 ± 1.7 versus 7.4 ± 2.8 IU/L), and the time required to reach peak levels of FSH was significantly longer in women than in men (27 ± 5 versus 14 ± 8 hours). The area under the serum level versus time curve tended to be smaller in women than in men volunteers (339 ± 105 versus 452 ± 183 IU/L × hours), but the difference did not reach statistical significance. Together these data suggest that recombinant FSH is absorbed from its intramuscular depot to a lower rate and extent in women than in men. In both sexes a relationship between serum FSH levels and body weight was apparent. During the experimental period, other hormones remained low at baseline levels or were only slightly increased.

Conclusion: *Our findings indicate that recombinant FSH is well tolerated and that it is absorbed from its intramuscular depot to a higher rate and extent in men than in women. After intramuscular administration, its half-life is in good agreement with that previously reported for natural FSH.*

INTRODUCTION

Human follicle-stimulating hormone (FSH) is a gonadotropic hormone produced by the anterior pituitary gland, whose primary function is regulation of follicular growth in females and of spermatogenesis in males. Hormonal response is accomplished via specific membrane receptors on granulosa cells and Sertoli cells, causing adenylate cyclase activation and thereby secretion and/or synthesis of various factors essential for target cell differentiation and gamete maturation (1, 2).

The FSH molecule has a dimeric structure of which both subunits are glycoproteins in nature. The 92-amino acid α-chain and the 111-amino acid β-chain have each two N-linked oligosaccharide chains presented as complex heterogeneous multiantennary structures (3). The variable degree of glycosylation, especially of sialylation, creates a spectrum of FSH isoforms with differences in charge, bioactivities, and elimination half-lives (4, 5).

The expression of human FSH in Chinese hamster ovary cells transfected with both subunit genes (6, 7) resulted in the synthesis of intact human FSH (recombinant FSH). The polypeptide backbone of recombinant FSH is identical to that of natural FSH, whereas recombinant and natural carbohydrate structures are closely related (8). The charge heterogeneity and bioactivity of recombinant FSH were confirmed by chromatofocusing, receptor displacement, and by in vitro and in vivo animal studies (9–11). In comparison with commercially available urinary gonadotropin preparations, highly pure (99.9%) recombinant FSH appeared to lack intrinsic luteinizing hormone (LH) activity and to exhibit a very high specific bioactivity (>10,000 IU/mg protein). These properties prompted the further development of recombinant FSH by means of clinical studies examining its pharmacokinetic and antigenic properties in humans. This first human exposure study was performed in gonadotropin-deficient male and female volunteers to assess the safety and tolerance and the pharmacokinetic and pharmacodynamic properties of recombinant FSH after a single intramuscular injection.

MATERIALS AND METHODS

Subjects and study design

Fifteen gonadotropin-deficient, but otherwise healthy, volunteers (8 women and 7 men) participated in this four-center study. The study protocol was approved by the local ethics review committees, and written informed consent was obtained from all volunteers. Nine subjects had panhypopituitarism, either primary (n = 3) or secondary (n = 6), due to surgical removal of a nonmalignant pituitary tumor. Five volunteers suffered from congenital isolated gonadotropin deficiency, and one volunteer was diagnosed as weight-loss-related hypothalamic hypogonadism. Autoimmunity was excluded by anti-nuclear and specific antirecombinant FSH antibody assays. Subjects receiving estrogen/androgen replacement refrained from this therapy, which started 1 week (oral therapy) or 3 weeks (intramuscular substitution) before injection up to 1 week after injection while appropriate thyroid and glucocorticoid therapy was continued. With the exception of one male volunteer, all subjects had a history of proven normal gonadal function; seven out of eight women had one or more deliveries, and one woman and six men subjects responded well to previous hormonal therapy.

Subjects received a single intramuscular injection of 300 IU recombinant FSH (Org 32489, CP 90073; NV Organon, Oss, The Netherlands) in 2 mL solvent in the upper quadrant of the buttock. Blood samples were taken just before injection and at 0.5, 1, 1.5, 2, 3, 4, 5, 6, 7, 8, 9, 10, 12, 16 (optional), 24, 48, 72, 96, 120 (optional), 168, 216 (optional), and 264 hours (11 days) after injection. Blood samples were centrifuged, and serum was stored in 0.5 mL serovials at −20°C until analysis. Serum was assayed for immunoactive FSH, immunoreactive and bioactive LH, testosterone (T), estradiol (E_2), and inhibin.

Safety parameters

Safety analysis included clinical observations, i.e., blood pressure, heart rate, and body temperature, as well as laboratory assessments like routine urinalysis (pH, protein, acetone, glucose, hemoglobin), blood biochemistry (sodium, potassium, chloride, bicarbonate, phosphorus, calcium, glucose, urea, creatinin, uric acid, alkaline phosphatase, alanine and aspartate aminotransferase, lactic dehydrogenase, bilirubin, protein, albumin), and hematology (hemoglobin, hematocrit, erythrocytes, differentiated leucocytes, thrombocytes).

Serum samples were analyzed for the presence of antirecombinant FSH antibodies using a sensitive radioimmunoprecipation assay and ^{125}I-recombinant FSH as a tracer. When testing a mixture of two mouse monoclonal antibodies (MCAs) raised against recombinant FSH and recognizing and α- and β-specific epitopes, the sensitivity of the assay was 0.5 pmol/L and the intra-assay and interassay coefficients of variation (CV) ranged from 4.3% to 9.6% and from 0.8% to 2.7%, respectively. The induction of antirecombinant FSH antibodies after recombinant FSH treatment was judged by comparing before and after treatment samples according to criteria, allowing a probability of a false-positive result of <0.1%. All serum samples were tested in duplicate, and the MCA mixture was used as a positive control in all experiments.

Hormone assays

Immunoreactive FSH and LH was measured by an immunofluorometric assay using the time-resolved fluoroimmunoassay technique and reagent kits 1244-017 for human FSH and 1244-31 for human LH (Delfia, Pharmacia, Woerden, The Netherlands). These two-site assays use a β-directed capturing MCA and an α-directed europium-labeled detection MCA. The assays were performed as described by the manufacturer using the Delfia instrumentation system and MultiCalc software (Pharmacia). Follicle-stimulating hormone and LH immunoreactivity was expressed in terms of the 2nd International Reference Preparation (IRP) of pituitary FSH (code no. 78/549) and the 2nd International Standard for pituitary LH (code no. 80/552). The sensitivity of immunofluorometric assay was 0.05 IU/L for both gonadotropins, and the intra-assay and interassay CV were below 4.8% and 4.3% for FSH and 4.7% and 7.5% for LH, respectively. The cross-reactivity of the FSH kit with LH was <0.08% and of the LH kit with FSH <0.01%.

Serum bioactive LH was measured in an in vitro mouse Leydig cell bioassay as described in detail previously (10). The sensitivity of this assay for serum samples using 2nd International Standard 80/552 as the standard was 2 IU/L.

Serum T and E_2 were assessed by radioimmunoassay (RIA) using a coat-a count T RIA (reagent kit TKTT1 DPC, detection limit 0.27 nmol/L; Diagnostic Products Corporation, Los Angeles, CA) and a double antibody E_2 RIA (reagent kit KE2D1 DPC, detection limit 11.6 pmol/L; Diagnostic Products Corporation). The intra-assay and interassay CV were <9% and 13% for the T assay and <4% and 5% for the E_2 assay, respectively.

Serum inhibin levels were measured by RIA using an antiserum (no.1989) raised against purified bovine 31-kd inhibin (12). Purified bovine 31-kd inhibin iodinated by the lactoperoxidase method was used as a tracer. The standard was a pool of human follicular fluid (FF; 280 U/mL) that was calibrated against a rete testis standard preparation of defined bioactivity. The immunoreactivity of 1 mU FF was equipotent to 0.121 pg recombinant human inhibin (Biotech Australia, specific in vitro bioactivity 51.060 U/µg protein using World Health Organization [WHO] standard 86/690 as the standard). The recombinant α-subunit of human inhibin exhibited complete cross-reactivity in this assay system. The standard pool, which was diluted in plasma from castrated subjects, provided dose responses parallel to the plasma dilution curves. The sensitivity of the assay was 28 U/L and the intra-assay and interassay CV were <10%.

Data analysis

The peak recombinant FSH concentration (C_{max}) and the time of its occurrence (T_{max}) were taken from measured serum level data. The area under the serum level versus time curve (AUC) after a single dose of 300 IU was determined by means of the trapezoidal rule from zero time up to infinity ($AUC_{0-\infty}$) under subtraction of the baseline. The elimination half-life ($t_{1/2}$) was calculated after baseline correction on the basis of increases of FSH concentrations measured between 72 and 264 hours after injection, using log-linear regression. Data are presented as mean ± SD unless stated otherwise. Curvefit coefficients (r) represent Pearson correlation coefficients. Comparison of age, height, weight, and body mass index (BMI) between male and female volunteers was performed by means of the Wilcoxon's test. Gender differences of bioequivalence were tested in a one-way analysis of variance (ANOVA). Differences were considered to be statistically significant if $P \leq 0.05$.

Table 1 Clinical characteristics of volunteers*

	Age (years)	Weight (kg)	Height (cm)	BMI (kg/m^2)	FSH (IU/L)	LH (IU/L)
Females (n = 8)	36 ± 3	67 ± 13	162 ± 12	26.1 ± 4.3†	0.54 ± 0.34	<0.17
Males (n = 7)	31 ± 7	62 ± 11	171 ± 13	21.3 ± 1.7	0.63 ± 0.57	<0.36

*Values are means ± SD.
†Significantly higher in females than in males.

RESULTS

Volunteers

The mean age, weight, height, BMI, and serum gonadotropin levels at screening are listed in Table 1. No significant differences between male and female volunteers with respect to age, height, or weight were found, whereas BMI values were higher ($P = 0.04$) for the female volunteers. During screening, serum FSH levels ranged between 0.12 and 1.08 IU/L in males and between 0.11 and 1.63 IU/L in females. Serum LH levels were either undetectable (<0.05 IU/L) or very low, resulting in individual levels between <0.05 and 0.40 IU/L in females and between <0.05 and 1.13 IU/L in males.

Safety and tolerance

A single injection of 300 IU recombinant FSH was well tolerated, and no drug-related adverse experiences were noted. Neither pain nor skin redness was observed at the site of drug injection. Comparison of before and after treatment safety variables, i.e. blood pressure, heart rate, body temperature, blood biochemistry, hematology, and urinalysis, revealed no changes of clinical significance. When screening volunteers for the possible induction of antirecombinant FSH antibodies, no post-treatment increases in ^{125}I-FSH binding were observed.

Pharmacokinetic analysis

Individual and mean delta increases of serum FSH after intramuscular injection of 300 IU recombinant FSH in seven male and eight female volunteers are shown in Figure 1. In all subjects, serum FSH levels were raised at 30 minutes after injection, and 13 out of 15 volunteers

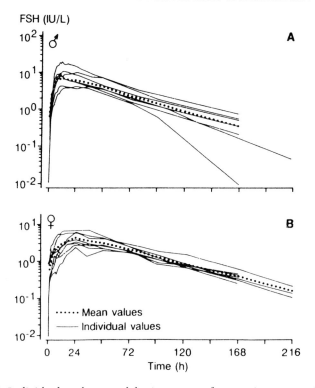

Figure 1 Individual and mean delta increases of serum immunoactive FSH after intramuscular injection of 300 IU recombinant FSH in seven men (A) and eight women (B) with hypogonadotropic hypogonadism

returned to baseline values 264 hours after injection. Individual pharmacokinetic parameters, AUC, C_{max}, T_{max} and $t_{1/2}$, are presented in Table 2. Within the group of male volunteers, one statistical outlier was identified by means of the Dixon test. This subject (M2), with an extremely low body weight (42 kg) and extremely high AUC value (876 IU/L × hours), was not included in mean values and was excluded from further statistical analysis. The mean $t_{1/2}$ of recombinant FSH was not significantly different between sexes (44 ± 14 versus 32 ± 12 hours). In contrast, C_{max} values were significantly ($P = 0.0072$) lower in female than in male volunteers (4.3 ± 1.7 versus 7.4 ± 2.8 IU/L) and T_{max} was also significantly ($P = 0.0004$) longer in females than in males (27 ± 5 versus 14 ± 8 hours). The mean AUC after administration of 300 IU recombinant FSH was 339 ± 105 IU/L × hours in females and 452 ± 183 IU/L × hours in males and thus tended to be lower in females, although the difference was not statistically significant ($P = 0.058$).

Table 2 Individual and mean pharmacokinetic parameters of recombinant FSH after one single intramuscular injection in the gluteal area in females (F) and males (M)

	AUC (IU/L × hours)	C_{max} (IU/L/h)	T_{max} (h)	$t_{1/2}$ (h)
F1	506	6.9	36	43
F2	255	2.8	35	35
F3	244	2.4	24	69
F4	252	3.1	24	40
F5	287	3.4	24	63
F6	292	3.8	24	33
F7	454	6.1	24	37
F8	425	5.9	24	31
Mean ± SD	339 ± 105	4.3 ± 1.7*	27 ± 5†	44 ± 14
M1	744	10.0	24	42
M2‡	876	18.4	10	40
M3	367	8.1	9	34
M4	599	10.9	10	44
M5	355	4.4	9	38
M6	250	4.1	24	12
M7	393	6.9	10	25
Mean ± SD	452 ± 183	7.4 ± 2.8	14 ± 8	32 ± 12

*Significantly lower in females than in males.
†Significantly longer in females than in males.
‡Statistical outlier not included in mean values.

Relationship between body weight and serum FSH levels

Comparison of body weight and serum FSH levels revealed a negative relationship in both men and women. Although the number of subjects studied are limited, the data suggest that there is a linear relationship between body weight and C_{max} values (males $r = 0.85$; females $r = 0.83$) and between body weight and AUC values (males $r = 0.89$; females $r = 0.86$). Scatter plots illustrating these associations are presented in Figure 2. The apparent linear relationships between BMI and C_{max} values (males $r = 0.48$; females $r = 0.61$) and between BMI and AUC values (males $r = 0.51$; females $r = 0.65$) were less strong (data not shown).

Other hormones

Serum LH levels were assessed during screening (see Table 1), just before injection, and at 1 and 3 days thereafter. Mean immunoreactivity

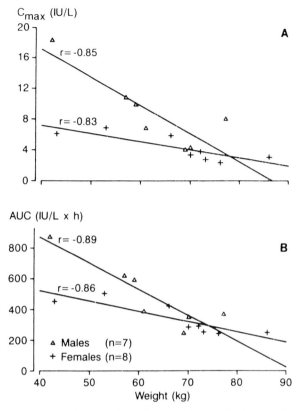

Figure 2 Correlation of C_{max} (A) and AUC (B) with body weight in seven men and eight women with hypogonadotropic hypogonadism

before and after treatment LH levels were below 0.4 IU/L for all subjects. Serum samples of five female and five male volunteers were also tested in the in vitro LH bioassay, but serum bioactive LH was below the detection limit of the assay (<2 IU/L) in all cases.

In females volunteers E_2 was detectable (>9.9 pmol/L) in only three women; 2 days after injection, two women showed a slight increase of E_2 (24 and 33 pmol/L, respectively). Serum inhibin was either undetectable (<30 U/L) or very low in female volunteers, whereas six out of seven males had detectable levels on inhibin. In comparison with baseline values, the mean inhibin of these six men was doubled (238±91 versus 124±66 U/L) 3 days after recombinant FSH injection. Serum T was either undetectable (<0.27 nmol/L) in two men or low (<10 nmol/L) in others, and no changes of any significance were noted (data not shown).

DISCUSSION

For nearly 30 years, infertility treatment with gonadotropins has been based on the application of crude urinary gonadotropin preparations, which have been proven safe and effective. The future of gonadotropin therapy, however, is likely to lie with highly pure recombinant human FSH preparations, devoid of other gonadotropins or inactive contaminants. Furthermore, FSH production by means of recombinant DNA technology is thought to guarantee an improved batch to batch consistency.

A general concern of recombinant glycoproteins is their potential immunogenicity. Because the peptide backbone structures of the natural and recombinant FSH were known to be identical, this concern was limited to possible minor differences in tertiary structure due to host cell processing. This first clinical study with recombinant FSH was performed in gonadotropin-deficient volunteers to minimize possible hazards in case of an antirecombinant FSH immune response and to prevent interference with endogenous gonadotropins. To date, many patients have been treated successfully with other recombinant glycoproteins, like erythropoietin, without developing specific antibodies (13). In the present study, no serum antirecombinant FSH antibodies were detected, but further studies will be required to demonstrate the safety of recombinant FSH during repeated administrations and long-term infertility therapy.

After intramuscular injection, the release rate of gonadotropins may depend on the formulation, injection depth, site, and volume (14). After intramuscular injection in the buttock, the absorption of immunoreactive recombinant FSH was very slow and even significantly slower in women than in men. Analysis of serum samples taken up to 72 hours after injection revealed that immunoreactive FSH levels were in good agreement with circulating bioactive FSH measured by an in vitro granulosa cell bioassay (Huhtaniemi I, personal communication).

Pharmacokinetic studies with urinary FSH and human menopausal gonadotropin (hMG) preparations administered via the intramuscular route have been limited but demonstrated previously that serum FSH levels depend on both the absorption and excretion rate of the drug. Diczfalusy and Harlin (15) reported that $t_{1/2}$ of hMG after intramuscular administration (>40 hours) is about four times longer than after intravenous injection. Daily injection of 150 or 225 IU urinary FHS in three women with isolated gonadotropin deficiency revealed a mean $t_{1/2}$ of 36 ± 16 hours, whereas $t_{1/2}$ varied between 33 and 59 hours in normal men after single intramuscular administration (160). The $t_{1/2}$ of recombinant FSH in the present study seems to be in good agreement with those reported for urinary FSH/hMG, although this is the first report on different release rates of FSH in men and women. Pharmacokinetic parameters like T_{max} and C_{max} are defined by the release of the drug from the intramuscular depot and by its $t_{1/2}$. However, the latter was not significantly different between the sexes; seeming differences may be attributed to the large intersubject variability. Sex differences in drug absorption and bioavailability after injection of aqueous solutions in the gluteus maximus, rather than in the vastus lateralus or deltoid, have been described previously and are thought to be related to the gluteal fat thickness, which is known to be greater in women than in men (14). Consequently, women may receive part of the drug in their subcutaneous adipose layer rather than intramuscular, leading to a less rapid absorption. Whether the latter also results in a lower absolute bioavailability, as indicated by the relative small mean AUC of the female volunteers, remains to be assessed.

Various studies support the hypothesis that body weight is a major determining factor on the dose and length of gonadotropin stimulation for induction of ovulation and for in vitro fertilization (17, 18). Follicle-stimulating hormone doses to initiate ovarian response may vary largely between individuals (19), and also thereafter major differences in ovarian response require close treatment monitoring. The present study revealed a strong negative correlation between body weight and serum FSH levels after recombinant FSH administration, thus suggesting that adjustment of doses of FSH in relation to body weight could reduce ovarian response variability.

In the current study, all volunteers, one man excepted, had previous proof of normal gonadal function. In view of its slow disappearance rate after intramuscular injection, a single injection of recombinant FSH might have been sufficient to induce temporarily gonadal response, influencing directly or indirectly the synthesis of other hormonal factors. During the experimental period, circulating immunoactive and bioactive LH levels were extremely low or undectable, as previously reported for patients with hypogonadotropic hypogonadism (20). Accordingly, serum T and E_2 levels were very low in male and female volunteers, respectively, and only two out of eight women showed a very small E_2 rise 2 days after injection. Follicle-stimulating hormone-induced E_2 synthesis, however, is known to be impaired in hypogonadotropic subjects (21–23), most likely because the minute amounts of residual LH are too low to support E_2 biosynthesis adequately. Interestingly, six out of seven men volunteers showed slightly increased serum inhibin levels 3 days after recombinant FSH injection. Using antiserum against bovine 31-kd inhibin, comparable levels of inhibin in men with hypogonadotropic hypogonadism were reported by others (24). The fact that no inhibin increases were observed in the female volunteers might be related to the relatively lower availability of recombinant FSH in these subjects.

In conclusion, the data of this first human exposure study with recombinant FSH (Org 32489, NV Organon) suggest that it is a safe drug with pharmacokinetic properties comparable with those previously reported for natural FSH. Further clinical data will be required to confirm the safety and efficacy of recombinant FSH in infertile patients treated for induction of ovulation or for induction of controlled ovarian superovulation.

ACKNOWLEDGEMENTS

We gratefully acknowledge Marc Roger, MD, and Najiba Lahlou, MD, Fondation de Recherche en Hormonologie, Fresnes Cedex, France, for the inhibin assessments and Renato de Leeuw, PhD, NV Organon, Oss, The Netherlands, for the gonadotropin and antirecombinant FSH determinations.

REFERENCES

1. Hsueh AJ, Adashi EY, Jones PB, Welsh TH. Hormonal regulation of the differentiation of cultured ovarian granulosa cells. Endocrinol Rev 1984;5:76–127.
2. Sharp RM. Intratesticular control of steroidogenesis. Clin Endocrinol (Oxf) 1990;33:787–97.
3. Boime I, Keene J, Galway AB, Fares FA, LaPolt P, Hsueh AJ. Expression of recombinant human FSH, LH, and hCG in mammalian cells: a model for probing functional determinants. In: Hunzicker-Dunn M, Schwartz NB, editors, Follicle-stimulating hormone: regulation of secretion and molecular mechanisms of action. Norwell, MA: Serono Symposia USA, 1990:120–8.
4. Ulloa-Aguirre A, Espinoza R, Damian-Matsumura P, Chappel SC. Immunological and biological potencies of different molecular species of gonadotropins. Hum Reprod 1988;3:491–501.
5. Ulloa-Aguirre A, Cravioto, A, Damián-Matsumura P, Jiménez M, Zambrano E, Díaz-Sánchez V. Biological characterization of the naturally occurring analogues of intrapituitary human follicle-stimulating hormone. Hum Reprod 1992;7:23–30.
6. Van Wezenbeek P, Draaier J, Van Meel F, Olijve W. Recombinant follicle-stimulating hormone I. Construction, selection and characterization of a cell line. In: Crommelin DJ, Schellekens H, editors. From clone to clinic, developments in biotherapy. Dordrecht, The Netherlands, Kluwer Academic Publishers, 1990:245–51.
7. Keene JL, Matzuk MM, Otani T, Fauser BC, Galway AB, Hsueh AJ, et al. Expression of biologically active human follitropin in chinese hamster ovary cells. J Biol Chem 1989;246:4769–75.

8. Hård K, Mekking A, Damm JB, Kamerling JP, Boer W, Wijnands RA, et al. Isolation and structure determination of the intact sialylated N-linked carbohydrate chains of recombinant human follitropin (hFSH) expressed in chinese hamster ovary cells. Eur J Biochem 1990;193:263–71.
9. De Boer W, Mannaerts B. Recombinant follicle-stimulating hormone II. Biochemical and biological characteristics In: Crommelin DJA, Schellekens H, editors. From clone to clinic, developments in biotherapy. Dordrecht, The Netherlands, Kluwer Academic Publishers, 1990:253–9.
10. Mannaerts B, De Leeuw R, Geelen J, Van Ravenstein A, Van Wezenbeek P, Schuurs A, et al. Comparative in vitro and in vivo studies on the biological properties of recombinant human follicle-stimulating hormone. Endocrinology 1991;129:2623–30.
11. Galway AB, Hsueh AJ, Keene JL, Yamoto M, Fauser BC, Boime I. In vitro and in vivo bioactivity of recombinant human follicle-stimulating hormone and partially deglycosylated variants secreted by transfected eukaryotic cell lines. Endocrinology 1990;127:93–9.
12. De Kretser DM, McLachlan DM, Robertson DM, Burger HG. Serum inhibin levels in normal men and men with testicular disorders. J Endocrinol 1989;120:517–23.
13. Watson AJ. Adverse effects of therapy for the correction of anemia in hemodialysis patients. Semin Nephrol 1989;9:30–4.
14. Zuidema J, Pieters FA, Duchateau GS. Release and absorption rate aspects of intramuscular injected pharmaceuticals. Int J Pharmaceutics 1988;47:1–12.
15. Diczfalusy E, Harlin J. Clinical-pharmacological studies on human menopausal gonadotrophin. Hum Reprod 1988;3:21–7.
16. Mizunuma H, Takagi T, Honjyo S, Ibuki Y, Igarashi M. Clinical pharmacodynamics of urinary follicle-stimulating hormone and its application for pharmacokinetic simulation program. Fertil Steril 1990;53:440–5.
17. Hedon B, Bringer J, Fries N, Thomas G, Pelliccia G, Bachelard B, et al. Influence of weight on the ovarian response to the stimulation of ovulation for in vitro fertilization. Contracept Fertil Sex 199;19:1037–41.
18. Chong AP, Rafael RW, Forte CC. Influence of weight in the induction of ovulation with human menopausal gonadotropin and human chorionic gonadotropin. Fertil Steril 1986;46:599–603.
19. Glasier AF, Baird DT, Hillier SG. FSH and the control of follicular growth. J Steroid Biochem 1989;32:167–70.
20. Dafau ML, Veldhuis J. Pathophysiological relationships between the biological and immunological activities of luteinizing hormone. Baillieres Clin Endocrinol Metab 1987;1:153–76.
21. Couzinet B, Lestrat N, Brailly S, Forest M, Schaison G. Stimulation of ovarian follicle maturation with pure follicle-stimulating hormone in women with gonadotropin deficiency. J Clin Endocrinol Metab 1988;66:552–6.
22. Shoham Z, Balen A, Patel A, Jacobs HS. Results of ovulation induction using human menopausal gonadotropin or purified follicle-stimulating hormone in hypogonadotropic hypogonadism patients. Fertil Steril 1991;56:1048–53.

23. Schoot BC, Coelingh Bennink HJ, Mannaerts BM, Lamberts SW, Bouchard P, Fauser BC. Human recombinant follicle-stimulating hormone induces growth of preovulatory follicles without concomitant increase in androgen and estrogen biosynthesis in a woman with isolated gonadotropin deficiency. J Clin Endocrinol Metab 1992;74:1471–3.
24. McLachlan RI, Finkel DM, Bremner WJ, Snyder PJ. Serum inhibin concentrations before and during gonadotropin treatment in men with hypogonadotropic hypogonadism: physiological and clinical implications. J Clin Endocrinol Metab 1990;70:1414–9.

Received July 7, 1992; revised and accepted September 16, 1992

This work was supported by NV Organon, Oss, The Netherlands

This paper was presented in part at the 39th Annual Meeting of the Society for Gynecologic Investigation, San Antonio, Texas, March 18 to 21, 1992

Correspondence: Zeev Shoham, Department of Obstetrics and Gynecology, Kaplan Hospital, Rehovot, 76100 Israel

8

Clinical outcome of a pilot efficacy study on recombinant human follicle-stimulating hormone (Org 32489) combined with various gonadotrophin-releasing hormone agonist regimens

P. Devroey*, B.M.J.L. Mannaerts[†], J. Smitz*, H.J.T. Coelingh Bennink[†] and A. Van Steirteghem[†]

*Centre for Reproductive Medicine, Academisch Ziekenhuis, Vrije Universiteit Brussel, Laarbeeklaan 101, B-1090 Brussels, Belgium and [†]Medical R & D Unit, NV Organon, PO Box 20, 5340 BH Oss, The Netherlands

ABSTRACT

In total, 50 couples participated in a pilot study evaluating the efficacy of various regimens of gonadotrophin-releasing hormone agonist (GnRHa) in association with recombinant human follicle-stimulating hormone (recFSH) in women undergoing in-vitro fertilization (IVF) and embryo transfer. The women were treated with recFSH alone (group I), or with recFSH in conjunction with pituitary desensitization using a buserelin intranasal spray, 4×150 μg per day, in a short protocol (group II) or in a long protocol (group III), or using triptorelin in a long protocol, giving a single dose of 3.75 mg i.m. (group IV) or daily s.c. injections of 200 μg (group V). In all women, treatment with recFSH resulted in multiple follicular growth and rises of serum inhibin and oestradiol. The latter indicates that the amount of remaining luteinizing hormone (LH) was sufficient to support FSH-induced oestrogen biosynthesis. On the day of human chorionic gonadotrophin (HCG) administration, endogenous LH was most profoundly suppressed in subjects treated with triptorelin. The median number of ampoules and treatment

This paper was first published in *Human Reproduction*, **9** (6), 1064–1069 (1994). Copyright 1994 Oxford University Press, reproduced with permission *days required in the various treatment groups varied from 21 to 36 ampoules and from 7 to 14 days, respectively. The median number of oocytes per group ranged from 9 to 11 and all cumulus–corona–oocyte complexes, with the exception of two, were classified as mature. The median fertilization and cleavage rates ranged between the treatment groups from 40 to 73% and from 73 to 100%, respectively. Fertilization failure of retrieved oocytes occurred in six couples with andrological or unexplained infertility. One patient had no transfer because of insufficient embryo quality. Finally, 43 couples had an embryo transfer and the median number of embryos replaced in each group was three per transfer. Clinical pregnancies were established in 10 women, two of whom had a miscarriage, resulting in eight ongoing pregnancies (18.6% per transfer) and the birth of nine healthy children. It is concluded from the current study that recFSH treatment is effective and safe for patients and their offspring.*

INTRODUCTION

The expression of human follicle-stimulating hormone (FSH) in Chinese hamster ovary cells transfected with both subunit genes has resulted in the synthesis of intact recombinant human FSH (recFSH) (Keene *et al.*, 1989; Van Wezenbeek *et al.*, 1990). In comparison with natural FSH preparations, purified (>99%) recFSH (Org 32489, Puregon®) has a very high specific bioactivity (~10 000 IU/mg protein) and lacks intrinsic luteinizing hormone (LH) activity (Mannaerts *et al.*, 1991). Phase I studies of recFSH in gonadotrophin-deficient male and female volunteers revealed that recFSH is safe and well tolerated, and that the elimination half-life of recFSH is comparable to that of urinary FSH (Mannaerts *et al.*, 1993). In gonadotrophin-deficient women, daily administration of recFSH induced multiple follicular growth up to the pre-ovulatory stage, whereas oestrogen and androgen concentrations in serum and follicular fluid remained very low as compared to those measurable in normally cycling women (Schoot *et al.*, 1992; Shoham *et al.*, 1993). These data indicate that in the absence of LH activity, production of androgens in the theca cell is diminished and insufficient aromatase substrate becomes available for oestrogen conversion in the granulosa cell. Although the significance of oestrogens for follicle development can be questioned, it remains beyond dispute that oestrogens are mandatory for other reproductive processes, e.g. inducing the mid-cycle LH surge, endometrial proliferation and cervical mucus production.

Current FSH/human menopausal gonadotrophin (HMG) therapy for the induction of controlled superovulation is frequently combined with gonadotrophin-releasing hormone agonist (GnRHa) treatment to prevent premature luteinization. After an initial release of LH and FSH, continuous use of GnRHa induces a reversible state of hypogonadotrophic hypogonadism. The suppressive potency of GnRHa is related to their structure–receptor interaction, elimination half-life, dosage and route of administration (Barron et al., 1982; Brogden et al., 1989). Most frequently, short-acting GnRHa is given daily by subcutaneous injection or nasal spray, whereas long-acting agonists can be administered intramuscularly or subcutaneously as a single injection (Loumaye, 1990).

This pilot efficacy study in women undergoing in-vitro fertilization (IVF) and embryo transfer was undertaken to evaluate whether recFSH therapy can be combined with GnRHa treatment, i e. whether the amount of remaining endogenous LH activity due to pituitary desensitization is suffcient to support recFSH-induced multiple follicular growth, steroidogenesis and related reproductive processes. Therefore various GnRHa/recFSH regimens providing various degrees of pituitary suppression, were applied: treatment with recFSH only, or treatment in conjunction with pituitary desensitization using a buserelin intranasal spray in a short or long protocol, or using triptorelin in a long protocol by two different dosages and routes.

MATERIALS AND METHODS

Patients

In total 50 out of 54 women of infertile couples completed this single-centre study up to oocyte retrieval, which was the study end-point. Two women became spontaneously pregnant before hormonal treatment was started; in one woman (group I) progesterone concentration was too high before starting treatment; one woman (group I) was discontinued because of a premature LH surge. The overall mean (±SD) age, body weight and height of patients who completed the study were 30.4 (±3.3) years, 58.6 (±7.7) kg and 164.8 (±6.4) cm, respectively. All women had normal ovulatory cycles, proven ovarian response to clomiphene citrate (Clomid; Merell Dow, Switzerland) and/or HMG (Humegon, Oss, The Netherlands) and were scheduled for IVF and embryo transfer. The study protocol was approved by the institutional ethical committee and written informed consent was obtained from all patients.

Study design

This study was an open, non-randomized pilot study in which subjects were treated for one treatment cycle only. After screening the patients were numbered consecutively and allocated to five different treatment groups. Group I ($n = 9$) was treated with recFSH only; groups II ($n = 9$) and III ($n = 11$) were treated with recFSH in conjunction with buserelin intranasal spray (Suprecur; Hoechst, Frankfurt, Germany), 4×150 µg per day, in a short protocol (group II) or long protocol (group III); groups IV ($n = 11$) and V ($n = 10$) were treated with recFSH in combination with triptorelin (Decapeptyl; Ferring, Malmö, Sweden) in a long protocol either by administering one single dose of 3.75 mg i.m. (group IV) or 200 µg daily s.c. (group V). GnRHa treatment was started on the first day of the menstrual cycle. Patients allocated to group I and II started recFSH treatment 2 days later (cycle day 3). In groups III, IV and V, recFSH treatment was started after ~14 days of GnRHa pre-treatment when pituitary down-regulation was established (see Results). RecFSH (75 IU/ampoule, Puregon®, Org 32489; NV Organon, Oss, The Netherlands) was administered once daily i.m. in the buttock. The daily dose of recFSH was fixed for at least the first 3 treatment days to one (group II), two (groups III, IV and V) or three (group I) ampoules. Thereafter, the daily dose was adjusted per patient based on the outcome of ultrasound and/or hormone measurements. In groups II–V ovulation was induced with 10 000 IU of human chorionic gonadotrophin (HCG) (Pregnyl; NV Organon, Oss, The Netherlands) when at least three follicles of ≥17 mm were detectable or earlier when serum oestradiol exceeded 300 pg/ml per follicle of ≥12 mm. In group I, HCG was administered when endogenous LH showed significant rises, indicating follicular luteinization and ovulation. Oocyte retrieval was performed by ultrasound-guided vaginal puncture and classification of cumulus–corona–oocyte complexes and embryos was performed as previously described (Staessen *et al.*,1989). At transfer a maximum of three embryos was replaced into the uterus and supernumerary embryos were cryopreserved. All subjects received luteal phase support by means of intravaginally administered micronized natural progesterone (600 mg/day; Utrogestan, Piette, Belgium) (Smitz *et al.*, 1992). Clinical pregnancies were defined as gestations with embryonic sacs, as identified by ultrasound; ongoing pregnancies were confirmed when positive fetal heart activity was detected 12–16 weeks after embryo transfer.

Ultrasonography and (anti)hormone assays

During each treatment cycle, transvaginal ultrasonography was performed at regular intervals to measure growth of individual follicles (≥12 mm). To monitor hormonal responses, morning blood samples were analysed for FSH, oestradiol, LH and progesterone by means of commercial assays as previously described by Smitz et al. (1988a). Inhibin concentrations on the first recFSH treatment day and on the day of administration of HCG were measured in 25 of the 50 patients by means of a commercially available enzyme immunoassay from Medgenix (Fleurus, Belgium). The antibodies of this assay crossreact with free α-subunits and with large precursor molecules (>33 kDa). The sensitivity of this assay was 0.6 U/ml and the intra-assay and inter-assay coefficients of variation were <10%. The induction of anti-FSH antibodies after recFSH treatment was judged by means of interaction with ^{125}I-labelled recFSH in a sensitive radioimmunoprecipitation assay as previously described by Mannaerts et al. (1993).

Statistical analysis

All statistical tests were two-tailed and carried out at the 5% level of significance. The comparison of groups was carried out using a non-parametric approach, i.e. the Kruskal–Wallis test was performed to detect significant differences in the five treatment groups and the Mann–Whitney test was performed for the two-by-two comparisons in cases of a global significant difference in the Kruskal–Wallis test.

RESULTS

Patient characteristics

In this open study, a comparison of age, weight and height did not reveal any significant differences between patients of the five treatment groups (Table 1). Causes of infertility were tubal (n = 21), andrological (n = 11), unexplained (n = 11) and endometriosis (n = 7). In total, 27 women suffered from primary infertility and 23 women from secondary infertility.

Table 1 Clinical characteristics of patients

	Treatment group[a]				
	I	II	III	IV	V
Number of patients	9	9	11	11	10
Age (years)	30.2 (±3.2)	27.7 (±2.1)	31.5 (±2.9)	30.9 (±3.9)	31.4 (±2.7)
Weight (kg)	54.7 (±6.3)	59.4 (±6.7)	59.5 (±8.7)	59.5 (±7.0)	59.3 (±9.4)
Height (cm)	164 (±7)	165 (±4)	164 (±8)	164 (±6)	167 (±8)
Cause of infertility					
tubal	5	3	5	3	5
andrological	–	2	5	4	–
endometriosis	1	1	–	1	4
unexplained	3	3	1	3	1
Parity					
primary infertility	4	6	6	7	4
secondary infertility	5	3	5	4	6

[a]Treatment in groups I, II, III, IV and V was respectively recFSH alone; recFSH + buserelin intranasal spray, short protocol; recFSH + buserelin intranasal spray, long protocol; recFSH + triptorelin, long protocol, single dose; and recFSH + triptorelin, long protocol, daily dose.

Table 2 Median (range) values of hormones measured at the first day of recFSH (groups I, III, IV, V) or 2 days prior to the start of recFSH treatment (group II) at the start of buserelin treatment

	Treatment group[a]				
	I	II	III	IV	V
FSH (IU/l)	9 (6–14)	6 (3–9)	4 (2–10)	3 (1–11)	4 (<1–7)
LH (IU/l)	6.7 (5.6–12.0)	4.9 (2.4–7.3)	3.2 (0.1–4.6)	2.8 (2.3–4.9)	2.4 (1.5–4.5)
Oestradiol (pg/ml)	39 (17–59)	33 (21–38)	33 (14–65)	27 (<15–34)	24 (<20–266)
Progesterone (ng/ml)	0.5 (<0.1–1.5)	0.4 (0.1–0.7)	0.2 (<0.1–0.8)	0.3 (<0.1–0.4)	0.1 (<0.1–1.0)

[a]See Table 1.
FSH = follicle-stimulating hormone; LH = luteinizing hormone.

Baseline characteristics

The median number of days required for pituitary down-regulation was 14 days in groups III, IV and V and ranged between 12 and 37 days of GnRHa treatment. Median baseline concentrations (and ranges) of FSH, LH, oestradiol and progesterone are presented in Table 2 and represent values measured on the first recFSH treatment day (groups I, III, IV and V) or values at the start of buserelin administration in a short protocol (group II). As expected, endogenous FSH and LH concentrations measured at menstrual cycle days 3 and 1 in groups I and II respectively were higher than those measured after 2 weeks of desensitization. After down-regulation with buserelin or triptorelin, median concentrations of serum FSH and LH were comparable and ranged between 3 and 4 IU/l and between 2.4 and 3.2 IU/l respectively. With respect to baseline values of oestradiol and progesterone, no differences were noted between the five treatment groups.

Treatment dosage and duration

In Table 3 the total number of recFSH ampoules, the number of treatment days required to induce multiple follicular growth and the calculated daily dose per group are presented. The median numbers of

Table 3 Median (ranges) values of total number of recFSH ampoules, treatment days and recFSH ampoules per treatment day

	Treatment group[a]				
	I	II	III	IV	V
Ampoules	21 (15–27)	22 (7–50)	36 (20–57)	35 (24–81)	32 (20–49)
Treatment (days)	7 (5–9)	12 (7–17)	14 (9–16)	14 (12–18)	13 (10–18)
Ampoules/day	3.0 (2.3–3.0)	2.0 (1.0–2.9)	2.7 (2.0–3.6)	2.6 (2.0–4.8)	2.5 (2.0–3.5)

[a]See Table 1.

ampoules used in patients treated with recFSH combined with a long protocol of buserelin or triptorelin in groups III, IV and V were comparable, i.e. 36, 35 and 32 ampoules, respectively, though a large interindividual variability was noted within each treatment group. The total amount of recFSH required in patients treated without GnRHa or with buserelin in a short protocol was considerably lower, i.e. 21 and 22 ampoules, respectively. For group I (without GnRHa) this result was explained by the fact that five out of nine patients showed rises of LH or progesterone during recFSH treatment and received HCG (10 000 IU) after only 5–7 treatment days. As a result, the median number of treatment days was only 7 days in group I, whereas this period was 12–14 days in the other groups. The calculated median daily dose was three ampoules in group I, two ampoules in group II and 2.5–2.7 ampoules in groups III, IV and V.

Ovarian stimulation

In all women, treatment with recFSH resulted in follicular growth. The total median number of follicles of ≥12 mm measured 8–72 h before HCG administration ranged from 7 (group III) up to 11 (group V). The median number of large pre-ovulatory follicles of ≥17 mm was 5.5 in group V, three in groups II and III, two in group IV and only one in group I.

Median values and ranges of hormones measured on the day of HCG administration are presented in Table 4. Serum FSH concentrations were

Table 4 Median (range) values of hormones measured in blood samples taken on the morning of the day of HCG administration

	Treatment group[a]				
	I	II	III	IV	V
FSH (IU/l)	21 (14–26)	13 (4–17)	15 (4–24)	17 (9–27)	17 (8–30)
LH (IU/l)	5.1 (1.2–20.0)	2.3 (<0.5–12.0)	1.3 (<0.5–7.1)	1.2 (0.8–3.5)	1.6 (<0.5–2.7)
Oestradiol (pg/ml)	1101 (684–2467)	1899 (948–2640)	1773 (711–2958)	1768 (781–2952)	1531 (893–3350)
Progesterone (ng/ml)	0.5 (0.2–1.6)	0.3 (0.2–1.3)	0.6 (<0.1–1.5)	0.5 (0.2–1.3)	0.9 (0.3–4.5)

[a]See Table 1.

highest in group I and lowest in group II with median daily doses of three and two ampoules of recFSH respectively (see above). Comparable concentrations of FSH were measured in groups III–V treated with a GnRHa in a long protocol. Median and maximal concentrations of circulating immunoactive LH reflected the degree of pituitary suppression due to various regimens applied, being most profound in subjects treated with triptorelin (Table 4).

No differences ($P = 0.6$) were noted between groups with respect to serum oestradiol concentrations. Serum progesterone concentrations were comparable between groups I–IV and higher in group V, which is in accordance with the larger number of preovulatory follicles of ≥17 mm noted in this group.

Inhibin concentrations, assessed in 25 out of 50 patients prior to the first recFSH injection and on the day of HCG injection, were increased in all cases. The overall median value of serum inhibin was 11.3 (2.3–23.1) IU/l after recFSH treatment versus <0.6 (<0.6–1.8) IU/l prior to the first recFSH injection.

Oocyte retrieval, embryo transfer and cycle outcome

The total number of oocytes retrieved and fertilization and cleavage rates are given in Table 5. The median number of oocytes retrieved ranged between 7 and 11 and was not significantly different between the treatment groups. All cumulus–corona–oocyte complexes were

Table 5 Median (range) number of oocytes recovered and fertilization and cleavage rates (%)

	Treatment group[a]				
	I	II	III	IV	V
Oocytes/ retrieval	7 (3–23)	9 (6–13)	11 (2–18)	10 (4–20)	11 (6–19)
Fertilization rate	64 (0–100)	64 (0–100)	73 (43–100)	40 (0–87)	62 (26–89)
Cleavage rate	73 (50–100)	90 (57–100)	78 (33–100)	85 (71–100)	100 (40–100)

[a]See Table 1.

classified as mature, with the exception of two embryos in groups III and IV, respectively. The median fertilisation and cleavage rates ranged between the treatment groups from 40 to 73% and from 73 to 100%, respectively. Attempts to fertilize oocytes failed in six couples with andrological ($n = 3$) and unexplained ($n = 3$) infertility. One patient had no transfer because of insufficient embryo quality. In total, 43 couples had an embryo transfer and the mean number of embryos replaced per group ranged between 2.3 and 2.8.

In group I no pregnancy was established, although one subject had a positive initial HCG test. In groups II–V clinical pregnancies were established in 10 women, two of whom had a miscarriage, resulting in eight ongoing pregnancies (18.6% per transfer) including one twin pregnancy (Table 6).

Pregnancy outcome

The ongoing pregnancies achieved were uneventful and nine healthy children, weighing (mean ± SD) 3087 ± 381 g, were born at a gestational age of 36 (twin) to 40 weeks. Extensive paediatric examination of the newborns revealed only minor malformations in the set of twins, i.e. one baby was diagnosed with mild hypospadias and the other with a torticollis. The latter disappeared within 10 weeks of kinesitherapy.

Table 6 Treatment cycle outcome

	Treatment group[a]				
	I	II	III	IV	V
Transfers	7	7	11	8	10
Miscarriage			2		
Single vital pregnancy		2	2	2	1
Multiple vital pregnancy		1			

[a]See Table 1.

Safety aspects

Daily i.m. injection of recFSH was well tolerated and was without induction of pain or skin redness. One woman who became pregnant after triptorelin/recFSH treatment (group IV) was hospitalized twice with the diagnosis of ovarian hyperstimulation, grade II. No other drug-related adverse experiences occurred. Anti-FSH antibody formation was not noted in any of the patients.

DISCUSSION

This is the first efficacy study of recFSH (Org 32489) in healthy women undergoing IVF embryo transfer (Devroey et al., 1993). The efficacy data show that recFSH stimulates normal multiple follicular development, as demonstrated by the number of preovulatory follicles, rises of serum inhibin and oestradiol and the number of mature oocytes recovered. The increases of serum oestradiol indicate that the amount of remaining endogenous LH, even after profound pituitary suppression with triptorelin, is still suffcient to support FSH-induced oestrogen biosynthesis. Thus, in IVF patients with normal regular cycles the amount of LH required (threshold concentration) is extremely low. Furthermore, the study data demonstrate the successful establishment of pregnancies regardless of the GnRHa regimen applied, and the overall ongoing pregnancy rate was comparable to that previously reported after stimulation with gonadotrophins of urinary origin (Smitz et al., 1988b, 1992). The case of one of the first patients in this study, allocated to group II, who was successfully treated with only nine ampoules of recFSH (675 IU) was reported previously as the first ongoing pregnancy and singleton term birth after ovarian stimulation with recFSH (Devroey *et al.*, 1992a,b). Another pregnancy obtained with GONAL-F® was published (Germond *et al.*, 1992).

The current pilot study did not intend to compare the success rates of different GnRHa/recFSH regimens. The number of observations was far too small and the inter-subject variability too large for this purpose. Comparison of ovarian responsivity due to treatment with recFSH alone, or with recFSH combined with GnRHa in a short protocol, with that induced by recFSH and GnRHa in a long protocol is complicated due to different baseline conditions of hormones and follicles at the start of recFSH therapy. Moreover, in the current study the starting dose of recFSH during the first 3 treatment days was fixed to three ampoules in patients treated with recFSH only, one ampoule (75 IU) in patients treated in the short protocol and two ampoules in those treated in a long protocol of GnRHa. Such treatment differences are likely to influence the initial selection of small antral follicles (Baird, 1987). Therefore, only the ovarian responses of subjects treated with buserelin (intranasal, group III) or triptorelin (i.m. or s.c., groups IV and V) in a long protocol are comparable, but the clinical outcome of these three treatment groups was very similar. The relatively low recFSH dose and short treatment period required in patients treated with a short protocol of buserelin, in which three out of nine patients became pregnant, illustrates the very favourable cost–efficacy ratio of this regimen.

In addition to actions on the anterior pituitary gland, GnRH and its agonists may exert direct effects on the ovary via highly specific GnRH receptors (Latouche *et al.*, 1989). It has been described previously that GnRHa may suppress FSH-induced cellular differentiation and steroidogenesis by impairing the expression of LH receptors and induction of aromatase activity (Parinaud *et al.*, 1988; Guerrero *et al.*, 1993; Testart *et al.*, 1993). Such direct inhibitory effects might also contribute in a longer treatment period and/or higher dose of (rec)FSH/HMG required to induce ovulation when combined with GnRHa administration in a long protocol.

In summary, the successful treatment of IVF patients with recFSH in conjunction with various methods of pituitary desensitization is promising, since in the current study GnRHa/recFSH therapy appeared to be effective and safe for patients and their offspring. However, further clinical studies on recFSH treatment combined with pituitary desensitization and in comparison to urinary FSH/HMG will be required to prove the long-term efficacy and safety of this new biosynthetic hormone preparation.

ACKNOWLEDGEMENTS

The authors wish to express their thanks to all members of the Brussels Free University Centre for Reproductive Medicine and to study co-ordinator Mrs A. de Brabanter and study monitor Mr G. Lathouwers for their skilful assistance. Ms L. Timmer is gratefully acknowledged for performing the anti-FSH antibody assay. This work was supported by grants from the Belgian Fund for Medical Research.

REFERENCES

Baird, D.T. (1987) A model for follicular selection and ovulation: lessons from superovulation. *J. Steroid Biochem.*, **27**, 15–23.

Barron, J.L., Millar, R.P. and Searle, D. (1982) Metabolic clearance and plasma half-disappearance time of D-Trp^6 and exogenous luteinizing hormone-releasing hormone. *J. Clin. Endocrinol. Metab.*, **54**, 1169–1173.

Brogden, R.N., Buckley, M.M.T. and Ward, A. (1990) Buserelin. A review of its pharmacodynamic and pharmacokinetic properties, and clinical profile. *Drugs*, **39**, 399–437.

Devroey, P., Van Steirteghem, A., Mannaerts, B. and Coelingh Bennink, H. (1992a) Successful in-vitro fertilization and embryo transfer after treatment with recombinant human FSH. *Lancet*, **339**, 1170–1171.

Devroey, P., Van Steirteghem, A., Mannaerts, B. and Coelingh Bennink, H. (1992b) First singleton term birth after ovarian superovulation with recombinant human follicle stimulating hormone (Org 32489). *Lancet*, **340**, 1108.

Devroey, P., Mannaerts, B., Smitz J., Coelingh Bennink, H. and Van Steirteghern, A. (1993) Clinical outcome and endocrine patterns in IVF patients treated with various GnRH-agonist/recFSH (Org 32489) regimens. Presented at the 9th annual meeting of the ESHRE, Thessaloniki, Greece, 27–30 June, 1993. Abstr. No. 34.

Germond, M., Dessole, P., Senn, A., Loumaye, E., Howles, C. and Beltrami, V. (1992) Successful in vitro fertilisation and embryo transfer after treatment with recombinant human FSH. *Lancet*, **339**, 1170.

Guerrero, H.E., Stein, P., Asch, R.H., Polak de Fried, E. and Tesone, M. (1993) Effect of gonadotropin-releasing hormone agonist on luteinizing hormone receptors and steroidogenesis in ovarian cells. *Fertil. Steril.*, **59**, 803–809.

Keene, J., Matzuk, M., Otani, T., Fauser, B., Galway, A., Hsueh, A. and Boime, I. (1989) Expression of biologically active human follitropin in Chinese hamster ovary cells. *J. Biol. Chem.*, **246**, 4769–4775.

Latouche, J., Coumeyrolle-Arias, M., Jordan, D., Kopp, N., Augendre-Ferrante, B., Cedard, L. and Haour, F. (1989) GnRH receptors in human granulosa cells:

anatomical localization and characterization by autoradiographic study. *Endocrinology*, **125**, 1739–1741.

Loumaye, E. (1990) The control of endogenous secretion of LH by gonadotrophin-releasing hormone agonist during ovarian hyperstimulation for IVF-ET. *Hum. Reprod.*, **5**, 357–376.

Mannaerts, B., De Leeuw, R., Geelen, J., Van Ravenstein, A., Van Wezenbeek, P., Schuurs, A. and Kloosterboer, L. (1991) Comparative in vitro and in vivo studies on the biological properties of recombinant human follicle stimulating hormone. *Endocrinology*, **129**, 2623–2630.

Mannaerts, B., Shoham, Z., Schoot, D., Bouchard, P., Harlin, J., Fauser, B., Jacobs, H., Rombout, F. and Coelingh Bennink, H. (1993) Single-dose pharmacokinetics and pharmacodynamics of recombinant human follicle-stimulating hormone (Org 32489) in gonadotropin-deficient volunteers. *Fertil. Steril.*, **59**, 108–114.

Parinaud, J., Beaur, A., Bourreau, E., Vieitez, G. and Pontonnier, G. (1988) Effect of a luteinizing hormone-releasing agonist (buserelin) on steroidogenesis of cultured human preovulatory granulosa cells. *Fertil. Steril.*, **50**, 597–602.

Schoot, B.C., Coelingh Bennink, H.J., Mannaerts, B.M., Lamberts, S.W., Bouchard, P. and Fauser, B.C. (1992) Human recombinant follicle-stimulating hormone induces growth of preovulatory follicles without concomitant increase in androgen and estrogen biosynthesis in a woman with isolated gonadotropin deficiency. *J. Clin. Endocrinol. Metab.*, **74**, 1471–1473.

Shoham, Z., Mannaerts, B., Insler, V. and Coelingh Bennink, H. (1993) Induction of follicular growth using recombinant human follicle-stimulating hormone in two volunteer women with hypogonadotropic hypogonadism. *Fertil. Steril.*, **59**, 738–742.

Smitz, J., Devroey, P., Camus, M., Deschacht, J., Khan, I., Staessen, C., Van Waesberghe, I., Wisanto, A. and Van Steirteghem, A.C. (1988a) The luteal phase and early pregnancy after combined GnRH-agonist/HMG treatment for superovulation in IVF and GIFT. *Hum. Reprod.*, **3**, 585–590.

Smitz, J., Devroey, P., Camus, M., Khan, I., Staessen, C., Van Waesberghe, I., Wisanto, A. and Van Steirteghem, A.C. (1988b) Addition of buserelin to human menopausal gonadotrophins in patients with failed stimulations for IVF or GIFT. *Hum. Reprod.*, **3**, 35–38.

Smitz, J., Devroey, P., Faguer, B., Bourgain, C., Camus, M. and Van Steirteghem, A.C. (1992) A prospective randomized comparison of intramuscular or intravaginal natural progesterone as a luteal phase and early pregnancy supplement. *Hum. Reprod.*, **7**, 168–175.

Staessen, C., Camus, M., Khan, I., Smitz, J., Van Waesberghe, L., Wisanto, A., Devroey, P. and Van Steirteghem, A.C. (1989) An 18-month survey of infertility treatment by in vitro fertilization, gamete and zygote intrafallopian transfer, and replacement of frozen-thawed embryos. *J. In Vitro Fertil. Embryo Transfer*, **6**, 22–29.

Testart, J., Lefevre, B. and Gougeon, A. (1993) Effects of gonadotrophin-releasing hormone agonists (GnRHa) on follicle and oocyte quality. *Hum. Reprod.,* **8**, 511–518.

Van Wezenbeek, P., Draaier, J., Van Meel, F. and Olijve, W. (1990) Recombinant follicle stimulating hormone. I. Construction, selection and characterization of a cell line. In Crommelin, D. and Schellekens, H. (eds), from Clone Clinic, *Developments in Biotherapy,* **1**, 245–251 (Kluwer Academic Publishers).

Received November 4, 1993; accepted January 27, 1994

Correspondence: P. Devroey, Centre for Reproductive Medicine, Academische Ziekenhuis, Vrije Universiteit Brussel, Laarbeeklaan 101, B-1090 Brussels, Belgium

9

Recombinant human follicle-stimulating hormone and ovarian response in gonadotrophin-deficient women

D.C. Schoot*, J. Harlin[†], Z. Shoham[‡],
B.M.J.L. Mannaerts[§], N. Lahlou[¶], P. Bouchard**,
H.J.T. Coelingh Bennink[§] and B.C.J.M. Fauser*

*Section of Reproductive Endocrinology and Fertility, Department of Obstetrics and Gynaecology, Dijkzigt University Hospital, Dr Molewaterplein 40, 3015 GD Rotterdam, The Netherlands, [†]Department of Obstetrics and Gynaecology, Karolinska Hospital, Stockholm, Sweden, [‡]Department of Obstetrics and Gynaecology, Kaplan Hospital, Rehovot, Israel, [§]Medical Research & Development Unit, NV Organon, Oss, The Netherlands, [¶]Fondation de Recherche en Hormonologie, Fresnes, France and **Service d'Endocrinologie et de Maladies de la Reproduction, Hôpital Bicêtre, Le Kremlin Bicêtre, France

ABSTRACT

Seven women suffering from hypogonadism due to previous hypophysectomy, isolated gonadotrophin deficiency, or Kallman's syndrome [median age 39 years (range 24–45)] volunteered to participate in a study to assess ovarian response following multiple-dose administration of recombinant human follicle-stimulating hormone (rhFSH; Org 32489). Baseline serum FSH and luteinizing hormone (LH) concentrations were 0.25 (<0.05–1.15) IU/l and 0.06 (<0.05–0.37) IU/l, respectively. Subjects received daily i.m. injections of rhFSH for 3 weeks (week 1: 75 IU/day, week 2: 150 IU/day, week 3: 225 IU/day). Blood sampling and sonographic investigations were performed on alternate days. Steady-state FSH concentrations were reached ~3–5 days after alterations of the doses administered. Maximum FSH concentrations were between 7.1 and 11.8 IU/l, whereas serum LH concentrations remained

This paper was first published in *Human Reproduction*, **9** (7), 1237–1242 (1994). Copyright 1994 Oxford University Press, reproduced with permission *unchanged. Due to absent follicle development and lack of a rice in immunoreactive inhibin (INH) (response failure possibly due to early ovarian failure or resistant ovary syndrome) in two subjects, analysis of ovarian response was restricted to five volunteers. Serum androstenedione levels showed no significant changes during rhFSH administration. Although serum immunoreactive INH concentrations reached normal late follicular values [659 (388–993)IU/l], serum oestradiol revealed only a minor increase [77 (18–210)pmol/l]. Moreover, growth of (multiple) ovarian follicles was observed up to pre-ovulatory sizes (>15mm) in these patients. It may be concluded from the present study that (i) rhFSH exhibits no intrinsic LH activity; (ii) rhFSH stimulation in hypogonadotrophic women resulted in an immunoreactive INH rise which was similar to that in normal women, whereas in contrast only a minor increase in oestradiol concentrations was observed (suggesting normal granulosa cell function and low availability of androgens as a substrate for aromatization); (iii) despite the minimal oestrogen increase, ovarian follicles developed normally to the pre-ovulatory stage.*

INTRODUCTION

Animal studies showed that recombinant human follicle-stimulating hormone (rhFSH) lacks intrinsic luteinizing hormone (LH) activity and exhibits a high specific FSH bio-activity as compared to urinary gonadotrophin preparations (Keene et al., 1989; Mannaerts et al., 1991). In order to assess safety and pharmacokinetic properties of this compound, a single-dose study was initially undertaken in hypogonadotrophic female and male volunteers (Mannaerts et al., 1993). Administration appeared to be safe and no anti-rhFSH antibody formation occurred. Multiple-dose rhFSH administration in hypogonadotrophic women provides the opportunity to study the effects of FSH alone, without the presence of endogenous or exogenous LH, on granulosa cell steroid and immunoreactive inhibin (INH) production and development of ovarian follicles. Information obtained may add to recent contentions based on case histories indicating firstly that LH is needed to provide the substrate for appropriate oestrogen biosynthesis (Schoot et al., 1992a), confirming that the classical 2-cell two-gonadotrophin concept (Fevold, 1941) is operational in the human, and secondly that follicles may fully mature without a concomitant increase in oestrogen concentrations (Rabinovici et al., 1991; Schoot et al., 1992a), suggesting differential regulation by FSH of steroidogenic and mitogenic activity during granulosa cell differentiation. This multicentre study describes

Table 1 Individual clinical and endocrine characteristics of seven hypogonadotrophic female volunteers: numbers 1–3 suffered from isolated gonadotrophin deficiency (IGD), number 4 from Kallman syndrome (KS) and numbers 5–7 from secondary panhypopituitarism (HX). All were participating in a multiple-dose study using rhFSH

Volunteer	Age (years)	Body mass index (kg/m^2)	Previous HMG response (+/–)	Testosterone (nmol/l)	Cortisol (nmol/l)
1	39	20.4	+	NA	471
2	39	23.9	+	89	190
3	38	23.6	+	93	430
4	24	24.2	NT	160	384
5	42	28.6	+	NA	498
6	45	22.0	NT	207	1200[a]
7	36	23.9	NT	230	536

[a]Above normal limits due to medication. HMG = human menopausal gonadotrophin; NT = no previous gonadotrophin treatment; NA = not available.

pharmacodynamic effects of daily injections (with weekly increments) of rhFSH in seven hypogonadotrophic women.

MATERIALS AND METHODS

Subjects and study design

Seven gonadotrophin-deficient, but otherwise healthy, female volunteers participated in this multicentre study. The study protocol was approved by the local ethics review committees and written informed consent was obtained from all participants. Three subjects suffered from congenital isolated gonadotrophin deficiency (IGD) and one from Kallman's syndrome (KS); the remaining three volunteers were diagnosed with secondary panhypopituitarism (hypophysectomy = HX) due to surgical removal of a non-malignant pituitary tumour (craniopharyngioma or adenoma). In the past, all three women with IGD had received gonadotrophins for induction of ovulation. All three showed a normal ovarian response and two conceived. The KS patient had not formerly received gonadotrophin treatment. Gonadotrophins were administered to one of the women who had previously had neurosurgery, resulting in a triplet pregnancy. For further clinical information on participating subjects see Table 1.

Autoimmunity was excluded by antinuclear antibody assays. All subjects refrained from oral oestrogen replacement therapy (starting 1 week before injection up to 1 week after the last injection), while appropriate thyroid and glucocorticoid therapy (if required) was continued in the HX volunteers (patients 6 and 7).

All subjects received daily i.m. injections of rhFSH [Org 32489 (CP090073); NV Organon, Oss, The Netherlands] during a maximum period of 3 consecutive weeks in an increasing dose regimen [week 1: 75 IU daily (= 1 ampoule), week 2: 150 IU daily, and week 3: 225 IU daily]; 75 IU of the compound was dissolved in 0.5 ml of solvent (150 IU in 1 ml and 225 in 1.5 ml) and injected at 24h intervals in the upper quadrant of the buttock. To reduce the risk of ovarian hyperstimulation, daily injections of rhFSH were discontinued when at least one ovarian follicle attained a mean diameter of 14 mm and/or serum oestradiol concentrations were >1200 pmol/l. Sonography (transabdominal or transvaginal, using 3.5–5 MHz probes) was performed every other day to monitor changes in endometrial thickness (Shoham et al., 1991), whereas growth of all individual ovarian follicles was measured (Pache et al., 1990).

Blood samples were taken on alternate days prior to the moment of rhFSH injection (days 1, 3, 5, 8, 10, 12, 15, 17, 19). Additional blood sampling was performed during the 3 weeks following discontinuation of rhFSH administration, or earlier if appropriate, using similar intervals (days 22, 24, 26, 29, 31, 33, 36, 40). Blood samples were centrifuged and serum was stored in 0.5-ml serovials at –20°C until assayed.

Safety analysis included clinical observations, i.e. blood pressure, heart rate and body temperature, as well as laboratory assessments (urine analysis, blood biochemistry and haematology). Serum samples were analysed for the presence of anti-rhFSH antibodies using a sensitive radioimmunoprecipitation assay and ^{125}I-recombinant FSH as a tracer, as published previously (Schoot et al., 1992a).

Hormone assays

Immunoreactive FSH and LH were measured by an immunofluorimetric assay (IFMA) using the time-resolved fluoroimmunoassay technique and reagent kits 1244-017 for human FSH and 1244-31 for human LH (Delfia: Pharmacia, Woerden, The Netherlands). These two-site assays employ a β-directed capturing monoclonal antibody (MCA) and an α-directed europium labelled detection MCA. The assays were performed as described by the manufacturer using the Delfia® instrumentation system and MultiCalc software (Pharmacia) (Mannaerts et al., 1993).

FSH and LH immunoreactivity was expressed in terms of the Second International Reference Preparation (IRP) of pituitary FSH (code no. 78/549) and the Second International Standard (IS) for pituitary LH (code no. 80/552). The sensitivity of IFMA was 0.05 IU/l for both gonadotrophins and the intra- and interassay coefficients of variation (CV) were <4.8 and 4.3% for FSH and 4.7 and 7.5% for LH, respectively. The cross-reactivity of the FSH kit with LH was <0.08 % and of the LH kit with FSH <0.01%. Serum testosterone and oestradiol were assessed by radioimmunoassay (RIA) using a coat-a count testosterone RIA (reagent kit TKTT1 DPC, detection limit 0.27 nmol/l) and a double antibody oestradiol RIA (reagent kit KE2DI DPC, detection limit 11.6 pmol/l; Diagnostic Products Corporation, Los Angeles, CA). The intra- and interassay CVs were <9 and 13% for the testosterone assay and <4 and 5% for the oestradiol assays respectively. In addition, intra- and interassay CVs for the androstenedione RIA (Diagnostic Products) were <8 and 10% respectively. Serum immunoreactive INH levels were measured by RIA as previously described (Lahlou et al., 1993), using an antiserum (No. 1989) raised against purified bovine 31 kDa INH. Purified bovine 31 kDa INH iodinated by the lactoperoxidase method was used as a tracer. The standard was a pool of human follicular fluid (280 IU/ml) which was calibrated against a rete testis standard preparation of defined bio-activity. The immunoactivity of 0.121 IU follicular fluid was equipotent to 1 ng of recombinant human INH [Biotech Australia; specific in-vitro bio-activity 51.060 IU/μg protein using World Health Organization (WHO) standard 86/690 as the standard]. The recombinant α-subunit of human INH exhibited complete cross-reactivity in this assay system. The standard pool, which was diluted in plasma from castrated subjects, provided dose responses parallel to the plasma dilution curves. The sensitivity of the assay was 30 IU/l and the intra- and interassay CVs were <10%.

Data analysis

Comparison of baseline and maximum hormone concentrations, and time interval to maximum immunoreactive INH and oestradiol elevation was performed by means of Wilcoxon's rank sum test. Changes in serum FSH concentrations were analysed in all subjects ($n = 7$). Due to the absences of follicle development and of oestradiol and immunoreactive INH serum concentration increases in two HX volunteers [(numbers 6 and 7), non-response possibly due to early ovarian failure or resistant ovary syndrome], analysis of ovarian response was restricted to the remaining five subjects. Data are presented as mean±SD, or median and range. Differences were considered to be statistically significant if $P < 0.05$.

RESULTS

Age and BMI (weight/height^2) of all volunteers was 37.6 ± 6 years (range 24–45) and 23.8 ± 2.5 kg/m^2 respectively (Table 1). Four women received rhFSH (numbers 2, 5, 6, 7) for 3 weeks whereas three women had to stop earlier because of ongoing follicle growth (patients 1, 3 and 4 on days 12, 16 and 18 respectively). None of the women exceeded the upper limit of serum oestradiol (>1200 pmol/l).

Median (range) serum concentration of FSH and LH prior to rhFSH administration in the overall group was 0.25 (<0.05–1.15) IU/l and 0.06 (<0.05–0.37) IU/l, respectively. Serum androstenedione concentrations appeared not to differ between the group with previous surgery [patients 5–7; 0.20 (0.08–1.16) nmol/l] and the gonadotrophin-deficient volunteers [patients 1–4; 2.68 (2.05–7.76) nmol/l: $P = 0.07$] (Table 2). Baseline concentrations of serum testosterone were not significantly different ($P = 0.06$) in the HX group (<0.38 nmol/l) as compared to IGD women [0.56 (0.36–0.89) nmol/l]. Initial oestradiol serum concentrations did not differ between both groups [21.9 (<5.1–37.7) pmol/l for IGD women versus: 5.1 (<2.3–14.3) pmol/l for the HX group], as shown in Table 3. Initial immunoreactive INH serum concentrations were low [IGD group: 31 (<30–149) IU/l; HX group: 30 (<30–89) IU/l].

As a result of similar daily dosages during 1 week, changes in serum concentrations of FSH appeared to stabilize after ~5 days (Figure 1). On the fifth day, following four injections of 75 IU rhFSH, steady-state serum FSH concentrations in seven subjects ranged between 1.5 and 4.2 (median: 3.3) IU/l. Steady-state concentrations of serum FSH on the fifth day of week 2 (150 IU/day; $n = 7$) varied between 4.0 and 8.5 (median 7.2) IU/l. Maximum FSH concentrations ranged between 7.1 and 11.8 (median 8.1; $n = 7$) IU/l (Table 3). Decline to baseline FSH levels occurred within 7–13 days after cessation of administration (Figure 1).

Maximum serum LH concentration during the period of rhFSH administration remained low [0.13 (0.05–0.47) IU/l] (Table 2). Peak androstenedione concentrations during rhFSH administration tended to be higher in the volunteers with IGD [3.70 (1.92–4.73) nmol/l], as compared to the HX group [0.27 (0.14–1.95) nmol/l]. No statistically significant difference ($P = 0.14$) was observed between baseline and maximum androstenedione concentrations. For serum testosterone

Table 2 Potential theca cell stimulation and maximum androgen response due to multiple-dose rhFSH administration in seven hypogonadotrophic female volunteers[a]

Volunteers	Luteinizing hormone (IU/l)		Androstenedione (nmol/l)		Testosterone (nmol/l)	
	Baseline[b]	Maximum[c]	Baseline	Maximum	Baseline	Maximum
1	0.37	0.38	4.23	4.14	0.36	0.43
2	0.06	0.08	?.31	3.26	0.55	0.64
3	0.23	0.47	2.05	1.92	0.57	0.50
4	<0.05	0.05	7.76	4.73	0.89	0.50
5	0.09	0.13	1.16	1.95	<0.38	0.52
6	0.06	0.08	0.20	0.14	<0.38	<0.38
7	<0.05	0.13	0.08	0.27	<0.38	<0.38

[a]See Table 1 for patient diagnosis.
[b]Baseline = serum level prior to rhFSH administration.
[c]Maximum = maximum serum level during study period.

Table 3 Granulosa cell immunoreactive inhibin and oestradiol production and follicle development in response to rhFSH administration in seven hypogonadotrophic female volunteers[a]

Volunteer	FSH (IU/l)		Immunoreactive inhibin (IU/l)		Oestradiol (pmol/l)		Follicle number[b]		
	Baseline[c]	Maximum[d]	Baseline	Maximum	Baseline	Maximum	<8 (mm)	8–13 (mm)	>14 (mm)
1	1.15	8.5	<30	659	32.3	210	0	8	9
2	0.56	11.8	<30	581	<5.1	77	0	2	1
3	1.07	10.1	31	659	37.7	140	0	4	1
4	0.25	7.1	149	388	11.6	49	–[e]	–[e]	1[e]
5	0.07	8.3	<30	993	7.6	112	20	3	0
6	0.10	8.8	30	69	14.3	18	2	0	0
7	<0.05	9.9	89	143	2.3	49	0	0	0

[a]See Table 1 for patient diagnosis.
[b]Number of ovarian follicles on the day of maximum rise in serum oestradiol concentrations.
[c]Baseline = serum concentration prior to rhFSH administration.
[d]Maximum = maximum serum concentration during study period.
[e]Measured by abdominal ultrasound.

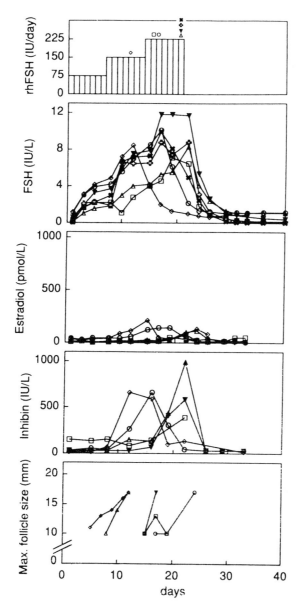

Figure 1 Daily dosage of recombinant human follicle-stimulating hormone (rhFSH). Upper panel: cessation of further rhFSH administration in three subjects is indicated and individual serum concentrations of FSH (IU/l), oestradiol (pmol/l) and immunoreactive inhibin (IU/l) in seven hypogonadotrophic female volunteers (shown by different symbols) participating in a multiple-dose study. Changes in sonographic size of the largest ovarian follicle (>10 mm) during rhFSH administration are indicated in the lowest panel

concentrations, no differences between groups or between baseline and maximum levels were observed ($P = 0.5$; Table 2).

Maximum serum oestradiol concentrations were reached [112 (77–210) pmol/l; $n = 5$] on day 19 (15–24). Maximum serum immunoreactive INH concentration was 659 (388–993) IU/l on day 15 (12–22). In all five volunteers with ovarian follicular development, the day of immunoreactive INH increase appeared to be significantly earlier as compared to onset of oestradiol increase ($P = 0.04$). In four of five subjects, immunoreactive INH dropped sharply just after discontinuation of rhFSH (Figure 1).

Initial transvaginal scanning of the ovaries revealed small follicles (<8 mm) in all the women of the IGD/KS group and one woman in the HX group (patient 5). No small follicles were observed in the remaining two HX women (patients 6 and 7). The presence of a single large ovarian follicle (at least one follicle ≥15 mm in diameter) was observed by ultrasound in four volunteers with IGD or KS during the second or third week of administration. Moreover, one woman showed development of more than five large follicles (patient 1). The rate of follicular growth in these patients appeared to be 2.1 ± 0.9 mm/day.

DISCUSSION

This study deals with multiple-dose rhFSH administration in seven hypogonadotrophic female volunteers, either due to the selective decrease of gonadotrophin biosynthesis (IGD or KS) or hypophysectomy (HX). The absence of endogenous and exogenous LH permits the study of the effects of FSH alone on ovarian steroid and INH production and follicle development. A discrepancy between oestradiol response and follicle growth in three of these women has recently been reported as case histories (Schoot et al., 1992a; Shoham et al., 1993). To examine the pharmacokinetic properties of rhFSH following i.m. administration, a single dose (300 IU rhFSH) study has recently been conducted in eight hypogonadotrophic women (Mannaerts et al., 1993). The observed T_{max} was 27 ± 5 h and $T_{1/2}$ was 44 ± 14 h.

From the present study it is clear that rhFSH exhibits no intrinsic LH activity since no rise in serum LH, androstenedione or testosterone concentrations (Table 2) occurred. rhFSH was administered i.m. daily, with weekly increments [from 1 to 3 ampoules (equivalent to 75 IU)/day]. The observed steady-state serum FSH concentration ~5 days was in agreement with the calculated half-life based on previous bolus studies. Maximum FSH concentrations as observed in the present study (median 8.8 IU/l) were of the same order of magnitude as perimenstrual concentrations in spontaneous cycles (Fauser *et al.*, 1993) and maximum serum FSH concentrations during gonadotrophin induction of ovulation according to a step-down dose regimen (Schoot *et al.*, 1992b). FSH stimulation resulted in an immunoreactive INH rise (median 659 IU/l) after 15 days which was similar to that in regularly cycling women (McLachlan *et al.*, 1987). In contrast, only a minimal increase in oestradiol (median 112 pmol/l) concentrations was observed following 19 days of rhFSH administration. This discrepancy in hormone biosynthesis by granulosa cells can be explained by the absence of androgen substrate, which is mandatory for adequate oestrogen production. Normal immunoreactive INH rise provides proof of normal granulosa cell function.

Immunoreactive INH is used as a marker for granulosa cell function in this study, but it should be noted that considerable doubt has recently been cast (Miro and Hillier, 1992) concerning its biological relevance. It should also be emphasized that two patients (numbers 6 and 7) have been excluded from the analysis of ovarian response, since an increase in serum immunoreactive INH and follicle growth as monitored by ultrasound was absent, presumably due to early (age 36 and 45 years) menopause, in these women.

To study the potential significance of androgen substrate availability further, subjects were divided into groups based on absent or intact adrenal function. Indeed, a difference in androstenedione and testosterone concentrations was observed when four individuals suffering from IGD/KS were compared with three women who underwent hypophysectomy. However, no difference was observed with regard to maximum oestradiol responses following rhFSH stimulation. In addition, no correlation between serum androstenedione and oestradiol concentrations was observed. This is not surprising, since androstenedione concentrations in follicle fluid (representing the amount of substrate available for aromatization within ovarian follicles) are 1000-fold higher (Pache *et al.*, 1992) and therefore minor differences in serum androstenedione concentrations may not influence local concentrations. Another intriguing observation is that the observed increase (doubling of baseline values) in immunoreactive INH started on day 12, whereas the minor rise in oestradiol concentrations began later on day 15. This difference was statistically significant ($P = 0.04$). It may be postulated that immunoreactive INH produced by granulosa cells may act as a paracrine regulator to stimulate theca cell androgen production, which in turn provides some substrate for oestradiol synthesis by granulosa cells (Hsueh *et al.*, 1986; Hillier *et al.*, 1991). A similar mechanism could be envisaged for changes in the intra-ovarian insulin-like growth factor (IGF) system, since it has been shown that

IGF1 is a potent stimulator of androgen synthesis by theca cells in culture (Hernandez et al., 1988; Magoffin et al., 1990; Bergh et al., 1993).

The present study clearly extends previous observations indicating that high intrafollicular oestradiol concentrations may not be a condition *sine qua non* for ongoing maturation of follicles. A discrepancy between serum oestradiol concentrations and follicle development has been observed when comparing urinary FSH and human menopausal gonadotrophin (HMG; with similar LH and FSH activity)(Couzinet et al., 1988) and combining urinary FSH with long-term gonadotrophin-releasing hormone agonist co-treatment (Remorgida et al., 1989). In addition, a case history has been published of a patient with 17α-hydroxylase deficiency who was therefore incapable of producing oestrogens (Rabinovici et al., 1989). Exogenous gonadotrophins induced growth of follicles up to the pre-ovulatory stage in this patient, and oocytes could be fertilized *in vitro*. Furthermore, fertilization and pregnancies were reported using rhFSH combined with gonadotrophin-releasing agonist in assisted reproduction (Devroey et al., 1993, 1994) and following induction of ovulation (van Dessel et al., 1994).

Puncture of three follicles (13, 15 and 18 mm in diameter) following rhFSH administration in subject 1 showed that both oestradiol and androstenedione concentrations within the follicles were indeed extremely low as compared to intrafollicular values in the late follicular phase under normal conditions (Schoot et al., 1992a; Pache et al, 1992). In the present study, four subjects exhibited extensive growth of at least one large follicle, whereas the number of medium-sized follicles also increased during rhFSH administration. However, in one patient (no. 5), follicle growth was disrupted even after increasing the daily dose of rhFSH. Although we feel that the physiological significance of this finding should be interpreted with great care, this study clearly demonstrates that follicles can be stimulated to grow to the pre-ovulatory size without a concomitant rise in oestradiol production. The assumption that FSH action at the follicular level largely depends on local up-regulation by oestradiol is mainly based on in-vitro animal studies (Kessel et al., 1985) and could not be operative in vivo in the human. In fact, so far there is doubt about the presence of oestradiol receptors within the human follicle, whereas androgen receptors have been clearly demonstrated by immunocytochemistry (Straus, 1992).

Although there is accumulating evidence that oestrogens are not mandatory for follicle development in the human, it is well established that under normal conditions oestrogen concentrations are strongly correlated with follicle size (Templeton et al., 1986). In line with these observations, it is believed that disturbed oestrogen production is responsible for cessation of follicle maturation in polycystic ovary syndrome patients (Franks, 1989). It may be speculated that under normal conditions next to FSH, other oestrogen-associated factors (such as changes in the inhibin or IGF system) are responsible for further stimulation of follicle growth, and therefore the rise in oestrogens is associated but not causally related to follicle development.

It may be concluded from the present study that rhFSH exhibits no intrinsic LH activity since a rise in serum androgen concentrations was absent. In addition, rhFSH stimulation in hypogonadotrophic women resulted in an immunoreactive INH rise which was similar to normal, whereas in contrast, only a minor increase in oestradiol concentrations was observed. This indicates norrnal granulosa cell function and insufficient availability of androgens as substrate for aromatization. Finally, despite the minimal oestrogen increase, ovarian follicles developed normally to the pre-ovulatory stage, confirming a dissociation between the mitogenic and steroidogenic activity of FSH.

ACKNOWLEDGEMENTS

The authors wish to thank D. M. de Kretser (Clayton University, Melbourne, Australia), D. M. Robertson (Prince Henry's Institute, South Melbourne, Australia), G. Bialy (National Institutes of Health, Department of Health and Human Services, Bethesda, MD, USA) and R. G. Forage (Biotech Australia Pty, E. Roseville, Australia) for the supply of reagents for inhibin radioimmunoassay. This work was supported by NV Organon, Oss, The Netherlands.

REFERENCES

Bergh, C., Carlsson, B., Olsson, J.-H., Selleskog, U. and Hillensjö, T. (1993) Regulation of androgen production in cultured human thecal cells by insulin like growth factor I and insulin. *Fertil. Steril.*, **59**, 323–331.

Couzinet, B., Lestrat, N., Brailly, S., Forest, M. and Schaison, G. (1988) Stimulation of ovarian follicular maturation with pure follicle stimulating hormone in women with gonadotropin deficiency. *J. Clin. Endocrinol. Metab.*, **66**, 552–556.

Devroey, P., Mannaerts, B., Smitz, J., Coelingh Bennink, H. and Van Steirteghem, A. (1993) First established pregnancy and birth after ovarian stimulation with recombinant follicle stimulating hormone (Org 32489). *Hum. Reprod.*, **8**, 863–865.

Devroey, P., Mannaerts, B., Smitz, J., Coelingh Bennink, H. and Van Steirteghem, A. (1994) Clinical outcome of a pilot efficacy study on recombinant human FSH (Org 32489) combined with various GnRH agonist regimens. *Hum. Reprod.*, **9**, 1064–1069.

Fauser, B.C.J.M., Pache, T.D. and Schoot, D.C. (1993) Dynamics of human follicle development. In Hsueh, A.J.W. and Schomberg, D.W (eds), *Ovarian Cells Interaction: Genes to Physiology*. Serono International Symposia Series, Springer Verlag, New York, pp. 134–147.

Fevold, H.L. (1941) Synergism of follicle stimulating and luteinizing hormone in producing estrogen secretion. *Endocrinology*, **28**, 33–36.

Franks, S. (1989) Polycystic ovary syndrome: a changing perspective. *Clin. Endocrinol.*, **31**, 87–120.

Hernandez, E.R., Resnick, C.E., Svoboda, M.E., van Wyk, J.J., Payne, D.W. and Adashi, E.Y. (1988) Somatomedin-C/ insulin-like growth factor as an enhancer of androgen biosynthesis by cultured rat ovarian cells. *Endocrinology*, **122**, 1603–1612.

Hillier, S.G., Yong, E.L., Illingworth, P.J., Baird, D.T., Schwall, R.H. and Mason, A.J. (1991) Effect of recombinant inhibin on androgen synthesis in cultured human thecal cells. *Mol. Cell. Endocrinol.*, **75**, R1–R6.

Hsueh, A.J.W., Dahl, K.D., Vaughan, J., Tucker, E., Rivier, J., Bardin, C.W. and Vale, W. (1986) Heterodimers and homodimers of inhibin subunits have different paracrine action in the regulation of luteinizing hormone-stimulated androgen biosynthesis. *Proc. Natl. Acad. Sci.* USA, **84**, 5082–5085.

Keene, J.L., Matzuk, M.M., Otani, T., Fauser, B.C., Galway, A.B., Hsueh, A.J. and Boime, I. (1989) Expression of biologically active human follitropin in chinese hamster ovary cells. *J. Biol. Chem.*, **246**, 4769–4775.

Kessel, B., Liu, Y.X., Jia, X.C. and Hsueh, A.J.W. (1985) Autocrine role of estrogens in the augmentation of luteinizing hormone receptor formation in cultured rat granulosa cells. *Biol. Reprod.*, **32**, 1038–1050.

Lahlou, N., Le Nestour, E., Chanson, P., Seret-Bégué, D., Bouchard, P., Roger, M. and Warnet, A. (1993) Inhibin and follicle stimulating hormone levels in gonadotroph adenomas: evidence of a positive correlation with tumour volume in men. *Clin. Endocrinol.*, **38**, 301–309.

Magoffin, D.A., Kurtz, K.M. and Erickson, G.F. (1990) Insulin-like growth factor-I selectively stimulates cholesterol side-chain cleavage expression in ovarian theca-interstitial cells. *Mol. Endocrinol.*, **4**, 489–896.

Mannaerts, B., De Leeuw, R., Geelen, J., Van Ravenstein, A., Van Wezenbeek, P., Schuurs, A. and Kloosterboer, H. (1991) Comparative in vitro and in vivo studies on the biological characteristics of recombinant human follicle stimulating hormone. *Endocrinology*, **129**, 2623–2630.

Mannaerts, B., Shoham, Z., Schoot, B., Bouchard, P., Harlin, P., Fauser, B., Jacobs, H., Rombout, F. and Coelingh Bennink, H.J.T. (1993) Single-dose pharmacokinetics and pharmacodynamics of recombinant human follicle-stimulating hormone (Org 32489) in gonadotropin deficient volunteers. *Fertil. Steril.*, **59**, 108–114.

McLachlan, R.I., Robertson, D.M., Healy, D.L., Burger, H.G. and de Kretser, D.M. (1987) Circulating immunoreactive inhibin levels during the normal human menstrual cycle. *J. Clin. Endocrinol. Metab.*, **65**, 954–961.

Miro, F. and Hillier, S.G. (1992) Relative effects of activin and inhibin on steroid hormone synthesis in primate granulosa cells. *J. Clin. Endocrinol. Metab.*, **75**, 1556–1561.

Pache, T.D., Wladimiroff, J.W., de Jong, F.H., Hop, W.C. and Fauser, B.C.J.M. (1990) Growth patterns of non-dominant follicles during the normal menstrual cycles. *Fertil. Steril.*, **54**, 638–642.

Pache, T.D., Hop, W.C.J., de Jong, F.H., Leerentveld, R.A., van Geldorp, H., van de Kamp, T.M.M., Gooren, L.J.G. and Fauser, B.C.J.M. (1992) 17β-Estradiol, androstenedione, and inhibin levels in fluid from individual follicles of normal and polycystic ovaries, and in ovaries from androgen treated female to male transsexuals. *Clin. Endocrinol.*, **36**, 565–571.

Rabinovici, J., Blankstein, J., Goldman, B., Rudak, E., Dor, Y., Pariente, C., Geier, A., Lunenfeld, B. and Mashiach, S. (1989) In vitro fertilization and primary embryonic cleavage are possible in 17α-hydroxylase deficiency despite extremely low intrafollicular 17β-estradiol. *J. Clin. Endocrinol. Metab.*, **68**, 693–697.

Remorgida, V., Veturini, P.L., Anserini, P., Lanera, P. and De Cecco, L. (1989) Administration of pure follicle stimulating hormone during gonadotropin releasing hormone agonist therapy in patients with clomiphene resistant polycystic ovarian disease: Hormonal evaluations and clinical perspectives. *Am. J. Obstet. Gynecol.*, **160**, 108–113.

Schoot, D.C., Coelingh Bennink, H.J.T., Mannaerts, B.M.J.L., Lamberts, S.W.J., Bouchard, P. and Fauser, B.C.J.M. (1992a) Human recombinant follicle-stimulating hormone induces growth of pre-ovulatory follicles without concomitant increase in androgen and estrogen biosynthesis in a woman with isolated gonadotropin deficiency. *J. Clin. Endocrinol. Metab.*, **74**, 1471–1473.

Schoot, D.C., Pache, T.D., Hop, W.C., de Jong, F.H. and Fauser, B.C.J.M. (1992b) Growth patterns of ovarian follicles during induction of ovulation with decreasing doses of human menopausal gonadotropin following presumed selection in polycystic ovary syndrome. *Fertil. Steril.*, **57**, 1117–1120.

Shoham, Z., Balen, A., Patel, A. and Jacobs, H.S. (1991) Results of ovulation induction using human menopausal gonadotropin or purified follicle-stimulating hormone in hypogonadotropic hypogonadism patients. *Fertil. Steril.*, **56**, 1048–1053.

Shoham, Z., Mannaerts, B., Insler, V. and Coelingh Bennink, H. (1993) Induction of follicular growth using recombinant follicle stimulating hormone in two volunteer women with hypogonadotropic hypogonadism. *Fertil. Steril.*, **59**, 738–743.

Straus, J.F. (1992) Does estradiol act as a local regulator of follicular growth and development? In *The Role and Uses of FSH in Induction of Ovulation*. Ares Serono, Geneva, pp. 11–21.

Templeton, A., Messinis, I.E. and Baird, D.T. (1986) Characteristics of the ovarian follicles in spontaneous and stimulated cycles in which there was an endogenous luteinizing hormone surge. *Fertil. Steril.*, **46**, 1113–1117.

van Dessel, H.J.H.M., Donderwinkel, P.F.J., Coelingh Bennink, H.J.T. and Fauser, B.C.J.M. (1993) First established pregnancy and birth after induction of ovulation with recombinant human follicle-stimulating hormone in polycystic ovary syndrome. *Hum. Reprod.*, **9**, 55–56.

Received October 11, 1993; accepted March 30, 1994

Correspondence: B.C.J.M. Fauser, Section of Reproductive Endocrinology and Fertility, Department of Obstetrics and Gynaecology, Dijkzigt University Hospital, Dr Molewaterplein 40, 3015 GD Rotterdam, The Netherlands

10

First established pregnancy and birth after induction of ovulation with recombinant human follicle-stimulating hormone in polycystic ovary syndrome

H.J.H.M. van Dessel*, P.F.J. Donderwinkel*,
H.J.T. Coelingh Bennink[†] and B.C.J.M. Fauser*

*Section of Reproductive Endocrinology and Fertility, Department of Obstetrics and Gynaecology, Dijkzigt Academic Hospital and Erasmus University, Dr. Molewaterplein 40, 3015 GD Rotterdam and [†]Medical R & D Unit, NV Organon, PO Box 20, 5340 BH Oss, The Netherlands

ABSTRACT

This case report describes the first established pregnancy and birth after induction of ovulation with recombinant human follicle-stimulating hormone (FSH) in a woman suffering from chronic clomiphene-resistant anovulation due to polycystic ovary syndrome (elevated serum luteinizing hormone and testosterone concentrations together with polycystic ovaries). Starting on day 3 of a progestagen withdrawal bleeding, 75 IU of rFSH was administered i.m. daily until a single preovulatory follicle was seen upon transvaginal ultrasound examination at day 13. Ovulation was induced by a single i.m. administration of 10 000 IU of human chorionic gonadotrophin, after which a viable singleton pregnancy was revealed at a gestational age of 6 weeks. The course of pregnancy and labour was uneventful and no abnormalities were found upon a paediatric examination.

This case report was first published in *Human Reproduction*, **9** (1), 55–56 (1994). Copyright 1994 Oxford University Press, reproduced with permission

CASE REPORT

A 27-year-old woman presented at our clinic with infertility of 3 years duration. A systematic work-up revealed evident signs of polycystic ovary syndrome (PCOS). Menstrual periods were irregular (8–52 weeks). Upon physical examination a body mass index of 25 kg/m^2 was found and moderate hirsutism was present. Hormone assays, 8 weeks after a progestagen withdrawal bleeding, revealed serum concentrations as follows: elevated serum luteinizing hormone (LH) (14.5 IU/l, normal range <8.6 IU/l); follicle stimulating hormone (FSH) (2.5 IU/l, normal range <7.0 IU/l); LH/FSH ratio 5.8; testosterone (5.1 nmol/l, normal range 0.5–3.0 nmol/l); and dehydroepiandrosterone sulphate (10.1 µmol/l, normal range 1.2–10 µmol/l). Upon transvaginal ultrasound examination the ovaries were noted to be polycystic (17 follicles in the right ovary and 23 follicles in the left ovary ranging from 2 to 7 mm in diameter). The volumes of the right and left ovaries were 24 and 20 ml, respectively, and the ovarian stroma showed enhanced echogenicity (Pache et al., 1992a). Hysterosalpingography revealed no abnormalities and sperm analysis was normal. Despite treatment with clomiphene citrate (up to 150 mg from cycle days 3–7) the patient remained anovulatory. Ovulation was successfully induced with human menopausal gonadotrophin (HMG) and adjuvant gonadotrophin-releasing hormone (GnRH) agonist during six cycles but no pregnancy was achieved. The patient subsequently agreed to participate in a multicentre study evaluating the efficacy of recombinant human follicle stimulating hormone (rFSH; Org 32489; Organon International bv, Oss, The Netherlands). The protocol of this trial was approved by the local ethics review committee. No GnRH agonist was provided. After induction of a progestagen withdrawal bleeding, i.m. injection of 75 IU/day (= 1 ampoule) of rFSH was started on day 3 and continued until day 13 (11 ampoules in total), which resulted in the development of a single dominant follicle of 18 mm diameter. All other follicles were <12 mm in diameter. Ovulation was induced by a single i.m. administration of 10 000 IU of human chorionic gonadotrophin (HCG; Pregnyl®, Organon) and confirmed by ultrasound 2 days later. For research purposes daily blood withdrawals and hormone assays were performed (Figure 1). The maximum oestradiol concentration concurrent with an 18 mm follicle was 660 pmol/l, within the normal preovulatory range for our laboratory (Schoot et al., 1992). Serum progesterone concentration 8 days following HCG was 28 nmol/l. No luteal support was provided. At 16 days after HCG administration the urinary test was positive. At 6 weeks amenorrhoea a singleton intrauterine pregnancy showing fetal heart beat was seen upon ultrasound examination. The ensuing pregnancy progressed without any

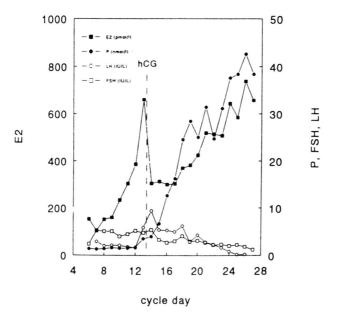

Figure 1 Daily serum oestradiol (E$_2$), progesterone (P) and follicle stimulating hormone (FSH) and luteinizing hormone (LH) concentrations measured by immunoradiometric assay throughout the treatment cycle with human recombinant FSH. The day of human chorionic gonadotrophin (HCG) administration is marked by the dotted line

problems. Antenatal check-ups were performed by a midwife (as is usual in the Netherlands in uneventful pregnancies). At term, spontaneous rupture of membranes with light meconium staining occurred, followed by an uneventful vaginal delivery (first and second stage 5 h and 30 min, respectively). A healthy 4600 g boy was born (Apgar score 7 and 9 at 1 and 5 min respectively). Paediatric examination revealed no abnormalities.

DISCUSSION

Recently, several reports of successful establishment of pregnancy and birth have been reported using rFSH for ovarian stimulation during in-vitro fertilisation (IVF) treatment (Devroey et al., 1992, 1993; Germond et al., 1992; Chuong et al., 1993). These studies show that rFSH can be used effectively to achieve the ovarian stimulation needed for IVF. However, induction of ovulation in clomiphene-resistant anovulatory women aims at the achievement of monofollicular development, which asks for a more subtle approach of compounds used, dose regimens and monitoring of ovarian response. This case history is suggestive of the utility of rFSH for this purpose by describing the first pregnancy and birth after ovulation using rFSH in a clomiphene-resistant, anovulatory woman suffering from PCOS. Earlier, we reported the achievement of pregnancy in this patient using FSH derived from recombinant technology resources (Donderwinkel et al., 1992).

The endocrine profile of patients suffering from PCOS is often characterized by high endogenous LH concentrations. High LH might be detrimental considering recent reports on a possible association between hypersecretion of LH and low conception and high miscarriage rates (Regan et al., 1990). FSH preparations derived from recombinant sources are devoid of intrinsic LH activity and, therefore, administration of these preparations might be particularly beneficial for PCOS women. However, it should be realized that, thus far, gonadotrophin preparations with low LH content have failed to show consistently improved results when used for induction of ovulation in PCOS patients (McFaul et al., 1990). Moreover, not all PCOS women exhibit elevated LH concentration (Fauser et al., 1992), and in this patient during rFSH administration LH concentrations were within the normal range (Figure 1), presumably due to preceding progestagen medication. It is of interest to note that in this patient normal pre-ovulatory follicle development and normal oestrogen production has occurred after low dose (1 ampoule/day) stimulation for 11 days resulting in FSH serum concentrations 8 IU/l. This is in favour of the concept of a low 'FSH threshold' in combination with normal selection of the dominant follicle in this patient (Pache et al., 1992b).

The present case shows that rFSH can be successfully used to achieve mono-ovulation leading to an uneventful singleton pregnancy and birth. Further clinical studies are needed to substantiate the efficacy and potentially beneficial properties of rFSH preparations for the induction of ovulation in clomiphene-resistant PCOS women.

REFERENCES

Chuong, C.J., Young, R.L., Boesch, C.L., Lewallen, N.B. and Reilly, M. (1993) Successful pregnancy after treatment with recombinant human follicle stimulating hormone. *Lancet*, **341**, 1101.

Devroey, P., Van Steirteghem, A., Mannaerts, B. and Coelingh Bennink, H. (1992) Successful in-vitro fertilization and embryo transfer after treatment with recombinant human FSH. *Lancet*, **339**, 1170–1171.

Devroey, P., Mannaerts, B., Smitz, J., Coelingh Bennink, H. and Van Steirteghem, A. (1993) First established pregnancy and birth after ovarian stimulation with recombinant human follicle stimulating hormone (Org 32489). *Hum. Reprod.,* **8**, 863–865.

Donderwinkel, P.F.J., Schoot, D.C., Coelingh Bennink, H.J.T. and Fauser, B.C.J.M. (1992) Pregnancy after induction of ovulation with recombinant human FSH in polycystic ovary syndrome. *Lancet,* **340**, 983.

Fauser, B.C.J.M., Pache, T.D., Hop, W.C.J., de Jong, F.H. and Dahl, K.D. (1992) The significance of serum luteinizing hormone measurements in women with menstrual cycle disturbances: discrepancies between immunoreactive and bioactive hormone estimates. *Clin. Endocrinol. (Oxf.),* **37**, 445–452.

Germond, M., Dessole, S., Senn, A., Loumaye, E., Howles, C. and Beltrami, V. (1992) Successful in-vitro fertilization and embryo transfer after treatment with recombinant human FSH. *Lancet,* **339**, 1170.

McFaul, P.B., Traub, A.I. and Thompson, W. (1990) Treatment of clomiphene-resistant polycystic ovarian syndrome with pure follicle-stimulating hormone of human menopausal gonadotrophin. *Fertil. Steril.,* **53**, 792–797.

Pache, T.D., Wladimimiroff, J.W., Hop, W.C.J. and Fauser, B.C.J.M. (1992a) How to discriminate between normal and polycystic ovaries. A transvaginal sonography study. *Radiology,* **183**, 421–423.

Pache, T.D., Hop, W.C.J., de Jong, F.H., Leerentveld, R.A., van Geldorp, H., Gooren, L.J.G., van de Kamp, T.M.M. and Fauser, B.C.J.M. (1992b) 17β-Oestradiol, androstenedione and inhibin levels in fluid from individual follicles of normal and polycystic ovaries, and in ovaries from androgen treated female to male transsexuals. *Clin. Endocrinol. (Oxf.),* **36**, 565–571.

Regan, L., Owen, E. and Jacobs, H.S. (1990) Hypersecretion of luteinising hormone, infertility, and miscarriage. *Lancet,* **336**, 1141–1144.

Schoot, D.C., Hop, W.C.J., de Jong, F.H. and Fauser, B.C.J.M. (1992) Growth patterns of ovarian follicles during induction of ovulation with decreasing doses of human menopausal gonadotropin following presumed selection in polycystic syndrome patients. *Fertil. Steril.,* **57**, 1117–1120.

Received July 28, 1993; acccepted September 17, 1993

Correspondence: H.J.H.M. van Dessel, Dijkzigt Academic Hospital, Room H 890, Dr. Molewaterplein 40, 3015 GD Rotterdam, The Netherlands

11

Recombinant human follicle-stimulating hormone and human chorionic gonadotropin for induction of spermatogenesis in a hypogonadotropic male

S. Kliesch, H.M. Behre and E. Nieschlag

Institute of Reproductive Medicine of the University, Münster, Germany

ABSTRACT

Objective: *To determine the efficacy of recombinant FSH administration to induce spermatogenesis.*
Design: *Case report, clinical study.*
Setting: *Tertiary center for reproductive medicine of the university.*
Patient: *A 44-year-old hypogonadal man with postpubertal pituitary insufficiency due to surgical removal of a prolactinoma.*
Interventions: *Recombinant FSH (150 IU three times weekly) was administered together with hCG (1,500 IU twice weekly). Control examinations were performed every 6 weeks, including hormone determinations, safety parameters, testicular volume measurements, and semen analysis.*
Main outcome measure: *Semen parameters.*
Results: *After 18 weeks of treatment, first sperm were seen in the ejaculate and reached normal sperm concentrations after 24 weeks of treatment. Serum hormone levels were in the normal range and testicular volume increased. No adverse side effects were observed.*
Conclusions: *Recombinant human FSH in combination with hCG can be used successfully for stimulation of testicular function in gonadotropin-deficient men.*

This communication-in-brief was first published in *Fertility and Sterility,* **63** (6) 1326–1328 (1995). Reproduced with permission of the publisher, the American Society for Reproductive Medicine (formerly The American Fertility Society)

INTRODUCTION

Fertility in men depends on both LH and FSH to induce androgen production and spermatogenesis. In hypogonadotropic hypogonadal men with GnRH deficiency or hypopituitarism, administration of urinary hCG and urinary hMG stimulates both androgen and sperm production (1). Recombinant human FSH was produced by Chinese hamster ovary cells that were transfected with the human FSH subunit genes. The purified recombinant human FSH showed pharmacokinetic and pharmacodynamic properties similar to natural human FSH (2). Recombinant human FSH, in contrast to hMG, is devoid of LH activity. Recombinant human FSH has been shown to be effective in ovulation induction and pregnancies were achieved after treatment with recombinant human FSH (3). In the male monkey recombinant human FSH increases serum inhibin levels as an indicator of Sertoli cell stimulation (4).

CASE REPORT

A 44-year-old hypogonadal man with pituitary insufficiency due to surgical removal of a prolactinoma was enrolled in a clinical trial to assess safety, tolerability, and efficacy of recombinant human FSH administered to induce spermatogenesis. The study was approved by the Ethics Committee of the University and written informed consent was obtained from the patient. At the age of 40 years, a macroprolactinoma was diagnosed, removed surgically, and, additionally, radiation was performed. Bilateral hemianopsia persisted and secondary hypogonadism was substituted by injections of 250 mg IM T enanthate every 3 weeks. Two clinical examinations were performed, both confirming hypogonadotropic hypogonadism and azoospermia. According to the medical history, pubertal development and development of secondary sex characteristics had been normal before the operation. Substitution therapy with T enanthate was terminated 6 weeks before first examination. Substitution therapy of pituitary function with corticosteroids, T_4, and vasopressin was continued as well as dopamine-agonist treatment to suppress hyperprolactinemia. During the treatment phase, control examinations were performed every 6 weeks. Serum levels of LH, FSH, and PRL were determined by highly specific time-resolved fluoroimmunoassays (DELFIA; Pharmacia, Freiburg, Germany). Testosterone and E_2 were measured by RIA. Testicular volume was checked regularly by palpation and ultrasonography. Semen parameters were analyzed according to World Health Organization guidelines (5). One hundred and fifty international units IM of recombinant human FSH (Org 32489; Organon International, Oss, The Netherlands) was given three times weekly (Monday, Wednesday, and Friday) in combination with 1,500 IU hCG (Pregnyl; Organon International) twice weekly (Monday and Friday).

RESULTS

Treatment lasted for 9 months and was terminated after induction of quantitatively normal spermatogenesis. During the study no side effects were observed. No induration or infection at the injection site occurred. After 18 weeks of treatment first sperm could be seen in the ejaculate. Serum hormone levels were in the normal range and testicular volume increased (Table 1). Sperm concentrations and sperm motility reached normal values while sperm morphology remained slightly subnormal (Table 1). α-Glucosidase, fructose, and zinc indicated normal function of the epididymis, seminal vesicles, and prostate (data not shown).

DISCUSSION

We report on the successful induction of spermatogenesis in a postpubertal hypogonadotropic hypogonadal man with hypopituitarism within 18 weeks of treatment with normal sperm concentrations attained after 24 weeks of treatment. The results indicate that treatment with recombinant human FSH is at least as effective in reinitiating spermatogenesis as hMG, if given in combination with hCG, with which first sperm may be seen in the ejaculate within 3 to 6 months of treatment in hypogonadotropic hypogonadism (1). Because of the mainly postpubertal status of the patients with hypopituitarism due to surgical removal of a tumor during adulthood, the reinduction of spermatogenesis is achieved effectively in these patients within several months (1).

However, as published earlier, the combined gonadotropin therapy has been shown to be as effective in GnRH-deficient males (1). Thus recombinant human FSH will be of use in these patients as well. Administration of recombinant human FSH was well tolerated without side effects. Thus, the availability of recombinant human FSH provides an effective and safe alternative to human urinary preparations. For safety reasons recombinant human FSH may help to avoid the potential risk of infections due to human origin.

Table 1 Hormone levels, combined right and left testicular volume, and semen parameters before and during treatment with recombinant human FSH

	Normal values	Weeks of treatment							
		−4	−2	6	12	18	24	30	36
FSH (mIU/mL)*	1 to 7	0.32	0.52	2.8	2.7	2.2	2.7	2.6	1.7
LH (mIU/mL)*	2 to 10	<0.12	0.36	0.62	<0.12	0.32	0.24	<0.12	<0.12
PRL (µIU/mL)*	<500	77	140	292	163	83	135	163	117
T (ng/mL)[†]	>3.46	1.13	1.04	6.52	6.87	3.40	5.05	6.12	5.31
E_2 (pg/mL)[‡]	<68	11.4	7.9	30.8	46.3	19.9	30.5	36.8	19.9
Testicular volume, right and left (mL)	≥24	17.6	19.1	22.0	22.0	23.4	27.0	27.0	28.0
Sperm concentration (×10^6/mL)	≥20	0	0	0	0	11.2	28.4	27.0	50.0
Sperm count (×10^6 per ejaculate)	≥40	0	0	0	0	44.8	122.1	102.6	110.0
Progressive motility (a+b) (%)	≥50					17	24	37	54
Normal morphology (%)	≥30					12	12	23	19

*Conversion factor to SI unit. 1.00.
[†]Conversion factor to SI unit. 3.467.
[‡]Conversion factor to SI unit. 3.671.

ACKNOWLEDGEMENTS

The technical help of Ms. Martina Niemeier, Ms. Christine Pix, and Ms. Giesela Tönnemann is gratefully acknowledged. We are grateful to Susan Nieschlag, M.A., for language editing.

REFERENCES

1. Kliesch S, Behre HM, Nieschlag E. High efficacy of gonadotropin or pulsatile GnRH treatment in hypogonadotropic hypogonadal men. Eur J Endocrinol 1994;131:347–54.
2. Mannaerts B, Shoham Z, Schoot D, Bouchard P, Harlin J, Fauser B. et al. Single-dose pharmacokinetics and pharmacodynamics of recombinant human follicle-stimulating hormone (Org 32489) in gonadotropin-deficient volunteers. Fertil Steril 1993;59:108–14.
3. Devroey P, van Steirteghem A, Mannaerts B, Bennink HC. Successful in-vitro fertilization and embryo transfer after treatment with recombinant human FSH [letter]. Lancet 1992;339:1170–1.
4. Weinbauer GF, Simoni M, Hutchison JS, Nieschlag E. Pharmacokinetics and pharmacodynamics of recombinant and urinary human FSH in the male monkey (*Macaca fascicularis*). J Endocrinol 1994;141:113.
5. World Health Organization. WHO laboratory manual for the examination of human semen and sperm–cervical mucus interaction. New York: Cambridge University Press, 1993.

Received June 2, 1994; revised and accepted December 28, 1994

Study medication was supplied by NV Organon, Oss, The Netherlands.

Supported by the Deutsche Forschungsgemeinschaft, Bonn, Germany (Ni 130/11)

Correspondence: Eberhard Nieschlag, Dr med., Institute of Reproductive Medicine, Steinfurter Straße 107, D48149 Münster, Germany (FAX 49-251-836093)

12

Efficacy and safety of recombinant follicle stimulating hormone (Puregon®) in infertile women pituitary-suppressed with triptorelin undergoing in-vitro fertilization: a prospective, randomized, assessor-blind, multicentre trial

B. Hedon*, H.J. Out[†], J.N. Hugues[‡], B. Camier[§], J. Cohen[¶],
P. Lopes**, J.R. Zorn[††], B. van der Heijden[†] and
H.J.T. Coelingh Bennink[†]

*Centre Hospitalier et Universitaire de Montpellier, 34295 Montpellier, [‡]Hôpital Jean Verdier, 93143 Bondy, [§]Centre de Procréation Médicalement Assistée, 80054 Amiens, [¶]Centre Hospitalier Intercommunal Jean Rostand, 923311 Sévres, **Hôtel Dieu, 40000 Nantes, [††]Clinique Universitaire Baudelocque, 75014 Paris, France and [†]Medical Research and Development Unit, NV Organon, 5340 BH Oss, The Netherlands

ABSTRACT

The objective of this study was to compare the efficacy and safety of a recombinant follicle stimulating hormone (FSH) preparation (Org 32489, Puregon®) with a urinary FSH preparation (Metrodin®) in infertile women undergoing in-vitro fertilization (IVF) and embryo transfer and who were pituitary-suppressed with triptorelin. In an assessor-blind, group-comparative, multicentre study, 60 women were randomized to Org 32489 and 39 to urinary FSH. An evaluation of the main parameter, the mean and total number of oocytes recovered, indicated a similar efficacy of the two preparations: 9.7 with Org 32489 versus 8.9 with urinary FSH. In addition, there were no significant between-group differences with respect to other efficacy variables such as the total dose used, length of treatment, number of follicles ≥ 17 mm in diameter and embryo quality. The ongoing pregnancy rates per attempt (30.2 versus 17.4%) and per transfer (34.0 versus 18.8%) were higher with Org 32489, but this difference was not statistically signifi-

This paper was first published in *Human Reproduction*, **10** (12) 3102–3106 (1995). Copyright 1995 Oxford University Press, reproduced with permission cant. No clinically relevant differences between Org 32489 and urinary FSH were seen with respect to safety variables. Serum antibodies were not detected in any of the subjects. It is concluded that Org 32489 compares favourably with urinary FSH in the treatment of infertile pituitary-suppressed women undergoing IVF and embryo transfer.

INTRODUCTION

Currently available follicle stimulating hormone (FSH) preparations are natural hormones derived from the urine of postmenopausal women and are used for the treatment of male and female fertility disorders caused by inadequate gonadotrophin stimulation of the gonads, and for controlled ovarian stimulation in medically assisted reproduction programmes. The clinical efficacy and safety of these preparations have been established. However, most urine-derived FSH preparations have a limited biochemical purity, ranging from 1 to 3%. In search of other sources of FSH, the development of a recombinant FSH preparation (Org 32489) was started. The expression of FSH in a Chinese hamster ovary (CHO) cell line transfected with both FSH subunit genes resulted in the synthesis of intact recombinant FSH (Keene et al., 1989; van Wezenbeek et al., 1990). The polypeptide backbone of Org 32489 is indistinguishable from that of natural FSH, whereas the recombinant and natural carbohydrate chain structures are closely related (Hård et al., 1990). The small structural difference does not affect the charge heterogeneity, receptor binding affinity and in-vitro and in-vivo bioactivity of Org 32489 (De Boer and Mannaerts, 1990; Mannaerts et al., 1991). In 1992, the first reports of pregnancy and birth of a healthy baby after treatment with Org 32489 for ovarian hyperstimulation with in-vitro fertilization (IVF) and embryo transfer (Devroey et al., 1992a,b) as well as for ovulation induction (Donderwinkel et al., 1992; Van Dessel et al., 1994) were published. Clinical studies performed since then have confirmed that Org 32489 is a safe and efficacious drug: studies in gonadotrophin-deficient volunteers have demonstrated that the preparation was well-tolerated, that anti-FSH or anti-CHO cell-derived protein antibodies were not observed, and that pharmacodynamic and pharmacokinetic behaviour of Org 32489 was similar to that of urinary FSH (Schoot et al., 1992, 1994; Mannaerts et al., 1993; Shoham et al., 1993; Matikainen et al., 1994). In addition, in clinical efficacy studies in ovarian stimulation followed by IVF and embryo transfer, treatment with Org 32489 proved to be a safe and efficacious regimen for both patients and their offspring (Devroey et al., 1994; Out et al., 1995).

The use of recombinant FSH offers advantages over urine-derived preparations, since the manufacturing process of a recombinant DNA technology product can be better controlled and an improved batch-to-batch consistency can be achieved. Furthermore, this new technology provides the opportunity to produce a highly purified product, which may result in a higher clinical tolerance and decreased risk of unwanted reactions with this preparation.

Current gonadotrophin therapy for induction of ovulation is usually combined with gonadotrophin-releasing hormone (GnRH) agonist treatment in order to prevent premature luteinization. In this study, triptorelin was used as the agonist because it has been demonstrated that with this drug a profound pituitary suppression can be achieved after s.c. administration (Porcu *et al.*, 1994).

The objective of our study was to compare the efficacy and safety of Org 32489 with a urinary FSH preparation in infertile women undergoing ovarian stimulation followed by IVF and embryo transfer, and who were pituitary-suppressed with triptorelin.

MATERIALS AND METHODS

Study design

The study was designed as a prospective, randomized, assessor-blind, multicentre trial. The study took place between August 1992 and July 1994 in six infertility clinics in France. A total of 100 subjects were planned to be included with a 3:2 ratio between subjects treated with Org 32489 and urinary FSH. Because, for technical reasons, Org 32489 was supplied in vials and urinary FSH in ampoules, a double-blind study design was not feasible. Instead, an assessor-blind design was chosen in which preparation and administration were performed by a study coordinator who did not take part in any decision concerning FSH administration during the study. The study was approved by a national ethics committee, and each subject had given written informed consent before participating in the study. The study was conducted in compliance with the Declaration of Helsinki and according to the European Community note on Good Clinical Practice for trials on medicinal products in the European Community (CPMP Working Party on Efficacy of Medicinal Products, 1990).

Selection of subjects

Inclusion criteria were: at least 18 and at most 39 years of age at the time of screening; a cause of infertility suitable for IVF treatment; a maximum of three previous IVF or other assisted reproduction attempts in which oocytes were collected at least once; normal ovulatory cycles with a mean length of between 24 and 35 days and an intra-individual variation of ±3 days; good physical and mental health; a body weight between 80 and 130% of the ideal body weight (adapted from the Metropolitan Life Insurance Company Tables).

Exclusion criteria were: infertility caused by endocrine abnormalities such as hyperprolactinaemia, polycystic ovary syndrome, and absence of ovarian function; male infertility defined according to $<10 \times 10^6$ spermatozoa/ml and/or <40% normal morphology and/or <40% normal motility; contra-indications for the use of GnRH agonists, FSH, human menopausal gonadotrophin (HMG), and/or human chorionic gonadotrophin (HCG); any ovarian and/or abdominal abnormality that would interfere with adequate ultrasound investigation; hypertension (sitting diastolic blood pressure ≥90 mm Hg and/or systolic blood pressure ≥150 mm Hg); chronic cardiovascular, hepatic, renal or pulmonary disease; a history of (within 12 months) or current abuse of alcohol or drugs (excluding smoking); and the administration of investigational drugs within 3 months prior to screening.

Study drugs and study procedures

GnRH agonist

Triptorelin (Decapeptyl®; Ipsen, Paris, France) was purchased locally in France and was given s.c. in a dose of 100 µg/day, starting on day 1 of the cycle.

Recombinant FSH

Recombinant FSH (Org 32489, Puregon®; NV Organon, Oss, The Netherlands) was supplied as a lyophilized powder in vials, each containing 75 IU FSH in-vivo bioactivity (batch nos. CP091077, CP091134 and CP092146).

Urinary FSH

Urinary FSH (Metrodin®; Ares-Serono, Geneva, Switzerland) was purchased locally in France and was supplied as a lyophilized powder in ampoules, each containing 75 IU FSH in-vivo bioactivity (batch nos. CP092047, CP092139, CP093057 and CP093107).

HCG

HCG (Pregnyl®; Organon) in a dose of 5000 IU/ampoule was purchased locally in France (batch nos. CP091122, CP092103 and CP092125).

Pituitary down-regulation with triptorelin was defined as serum oestradiol concentration <50 pg/ml and was to be achieved within 5 weeks maximally. Subsequently, treatment with Org 32489 or urinary FSH i.m. was started with a dose between 150 and 225 IU/day during treatment days 1–4. From treatment day 5 onwards, an individual adjustment was made according to follicular development, as assessed by ultrasound scanning. HCG (10 000 IU) was administered to induce ovulation when at least three follicles ≥17 mm in diameter were present. Embryo transfer was performed within 2 days of sperm/oocyte incubation and no more than three embryos were to be replaced. Luteal support was given during at least 2 weeks and included a minimum of three injections of locally purchased HCG (1500 IU) or at least 50 mg progesterone daily i.m. or 400 mg progesterone daily intravaginally.

End points

Because the aim of ovarian stimulation is to increase the number of oocytes available for fertilization, the primary parameter investigated in this study was the total number of oocytes retrieved per patient. Secondary end points included the total dose used, the duration of FSH treatment, the number of follicles ≥17 mm in diameter, the number of follicles ≥15 mm in diameter, the number of high quality embryos, the clinical pregnancy rate (i.e. urinary HCG >1000 IU/l and/or gestational sac on ultrasound) per attempt and per transfer, and the ongoing pregnancy rate (i.e. proof of a vital pregnancy continuing at least 12 weeks after embryo transfer) per attempt and per transfer.

The implantation rate was defined as the number of vital fetuses, as assessed by ultrasound at least 12 weeks after embryo transfer, divided by the number of embryos transferred for each subject.

The main safety parameters were the incidence of ovarian hyperstimulation syndrome (OHSS) and the development of anti-FSH and anti-CHO cell-derived protein antibodies, the latter being measured in serum before and after the treatment cycle, according to the methodology published previously (Out *et al.*, 1995). In addition, routine laboratory parameters were measured before and after treatment. These parameters included blood biochemistry such as sodium, potassium, chloride, bicarbonate, phosphorus, calcium, glucose, urea, creatinine, alkaline phosphatase, total bilirubin, alanine aminotransferase, aspartase aminotransferase, lactate dehydrogenase, total protein and albumin concentrations; haematology parameters, including haemoglobin, haematocrit, red blood cell count, white blood cell count plus differentiation and platelet count; urine analysis including pH, total protein, acetone, glucose and haemoglobin.

Evaluation methods

At screening, a medical history was obtained and a physical and gynaecological examination was performed. In addition to routine laboratory parameters, endocrinological parameters such as serum oestradiol, progesterone, FSH, luteinizing hormone (LH), prolactin, testosterone and dehydroepiandrosterone sulphate were also measured. An ultrasound scan was performed to exclude ovarian abnormalities and the spermatozoa of the partner was analysed. To measure follicular development, ovarian ultrasound scanning was performed on the first FSH treatment day prior to FSH injection, or 1–3 days prior to that first treatment day to demonstrate the absence of follicular structures ≥20 mm in diameter. Subsequent scanning was performed on days 4–6 of treatment, if feasible, and on a regular basis from day 8 of treatment onwards until the HCG injection. Assessments of serum oestradiol, progesterone, FSH and LH concentrations were performed on the first FSH treatment day prior to the FSH injection, or 1–3 days before that first day, and at the day of HCG injection or 1–3 days prior to that day. In addition, serum oestradiol and LH concentrations were performed according to local methods on days 4–6 of treatment, if feasible, and on a regular basis from day 8 onwards. The classification of oocytes as either mature or immature and of embryos as type 1, 2, 3 or 4 was carried out according to criteria published previously (Staessen et al., 1989). Type 1 and 2 embryos were classified as high quality embryos.

Statistical analysis

Analyses were based on 57 (out of 60 randomized) patients treated with ORG 32489 and 33 (out of 39 randomized) patients treated with urinary FSH. For non-dichotomous data analyses of variance were performed; if not applicable, the Wilcoxon test statistic adjusting for centre, or equivalently, the Mantel–Haenszel test statistic extended for multiple centres using standardized midrank scores per centre, was used. A parametric analysis based on Cochran and Whitehead's methods of combining individual centre results, was applied and used for

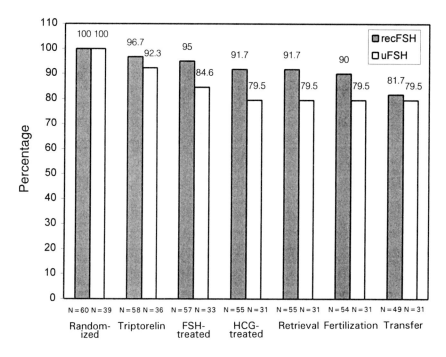

Figure 1 Disposition of subjects. recFSH = recombinant follicle stimulating hormone (Org 32489); uFSH = urinary FSH

the communication of results and eventual analysis alongside the Wilcoxon results (Whitehead and Whitehead, 1991). This approach meant that centres with the lowest SE of the estimate of the treatment difference received the highest weight in the analysis, thereby accounting for differences in the sample size per centre. For binary data, the Mantel–Haenszel test statistic extended for multiple centres was used.

RESULTS

Study population

A total of 99 subjects from six centres were randomized to the Org 32489 and urinary FSH treatments in a 3:2 ratio. In all, 60 subjects were allocated to Org 32489 and 39 to urinary FSH. A complete overview of the disposition of subjects is presented in Figure 1.

The number of subjects treated per centre ranged from three to 32. Both groups were comparable in demographic and infertility characteristics (Table 1). Tubal factor was the most frequent cause of infertility

Table 1 Main demographic and infertility baseline characteristics

Characteristic	Recombinant FSH (n = 57)	Urinary FSH (n = 33)
Mean±SD age (years, range)	32.2±4.1 (22–39)	31.2±4.0 (23–39)
Mean±SD height (cm, range)	162.1±5.8 (150–171)	164.6±5.4 (151–174)
Mean±SD weight (kg, range)	59.3±9.7 (45–100)	62.0±9.8 (48–91)
Mean±SD body mass index (kg/m^2, range)	22.5±3.3 (18.0–34.6)	23.0±3.8 (17.3–34.3)
Mean±SD duration of infertility (years, range)	5.4±3.1 (1–15)	3.7±1.9 (1–8)
No. of subjects with primary infertility (%)	19 (33.3)	11 (33.3)
No. of subjects with secondary infertility (%)	38 (66.7)	22 (66.7)
No. of subjects with cause of infertility (%)		
tubal disease	35 (61.4)	22 (66.7)
endometriosis	7 (12.3)	2 (6.1)
tubal disease/endometriosis	2 (3.5)	2 (6.1)
unknown	13 (22.8)	7 (21.2)

FSH = follicle stimulating hormone.

reported in both groups, followed by the category 'unknown'. In both treatment groups one-third of the subjects had primary infertility and two-thirds had secondary infertility. The mean duration of infertility for the Org 32489 and urinary FSH groups was 5.4 and 3.7 years respectively.

Clinical efficacy

The results on the efficacy parameters (all adjusted for centre) are presented in Table 2. The primary efficacy parameter, the mean total number of oocytes per retrieval, was 9.7 oocytes in the Org 32489 group and 8.9 oocytes in the urinary FSH group. The difference between the two treatment groups was 0.8 oocytes in favour of Org 32489, which was not statistically significant ($P = 0.53$).

With respect to the secondary efficacy parameters, the mean number of mature oocytes was also higher with Org 32489 treament compared with urinary FSH (8.1 versus 6.9 oocytes), as were the total dose used and all measures of pregnancy rate. None of the between-group differ-

Table 2 Primary and secondary efficacy parameters

Parameter	Mean adjusted for centre		P value	95% confidence interval[a]	SE[b]
	Recombinant FSH	Urinary FSH			
Primary efficacy parameter					
No. of oocytes retrieved	9.7	8.9	0.53	–1.7 to 3.2	1.3
Secondary efficacy parameters					
No. of mature oocytes retrieved	8.1	6.9	0.31	–1.1 to 3.4	1.2
Total dose used (IU)	2265	2213	0.75	–240 to 330	143
Duration of treatment (days)	10.2	10.3	0.83	–0.8 to 0.7	0.4
No. follicles ≥17 mm in diameter	5.4	5.5	0.84	–1.2 to 0.9	0.5
No. follicles ≥15 mm in diameter	7.3	7.2	0.83	–1.2 to 1.5	0.7
No. of high quality embryos	3.7	4.0	0.69	–1.7 to 1.1	0.7
Clinical pregnancy rate per attempt (%)	35.4	26.6	0.41	–12.1 to 29.6	10.7
Clinical pregnancy rate per transfer (%)	40.8	28.6	0.29	–10.3 to 34.8	11.5
Ongoing pregnancy rate per attempt (%)	30.2	17.4	0.19	–6.4 to 31.9	9.8
Ongoing pregnancy rate per transfer (%)	34.0	18.8	0.15	–5.5 to 35.9	10.6

FSH = follicle stimulating hormone.
[a]95% confidence interval of the estimated treatment difference.
[b]standard error of the estimated treatment difference.

ences in secondary efficacy parameters appeared to be statistically significant (Table 2).

There were no marked differences between the treatment groups with respect to endocrinological and biochemical parameters at the start of the treatment. On the day of HCG administration, the subjects in the Org 32489 group seemed to have higher median serum concentrations of oestradiol than those in the urinary FSH group (Table 3).

Table 3 Median (range, SD) endocrinological serum parameters

Parameter	Baseline					Day of HCG injection			
	n	Recombinant FSH	n	Urinary FSH	n	Recombinant FSH	n	Urinary FSH
Oestradiol (pmol/l)	44	91.8 (35.2–275.3, 53.6)	30	91.8 (18.4–212.9, 37.1)	50	7551 (1406–27 077, 5921)	28	5514 (165–12 665, 3062)
Progesterone (nmol/l)	35	0.6 (0.1–4.0, 0.7)	26	0.8 (0.1–13.5, 2.6)	43	1.4 (0.1–7.7, 1.9)	24	0.9 (0.3–5.8, 1.4)
FSH (IU/l)	29	5.1 (0.8–23.4, 3.9)	18	4.5 (3.0–8.9, 1.8)	37	13.9 (5.1–30.5, 6.9)	20	13.2 (2.2–30.0, 7.7)
Luteinizing hormone (IU/l)	45	2.0 (0.3–10.5, 1.7)	30	2.0 (0.5–6.8, 1.5)	50	1.5 (0.2–4.0, 0.9)	28	1.6 (0.7–4.0, 0.7)

FSH = follicle stimulating hormone.

Safety

Three subjects in the Org 32489 group were hospitalized with OHSS; two of them had an ongoing pregnancy. One subject in the urinary FSH group reported abdominal pain leading to hospitalization. All four subjects had an uneventful and complete recovery. The number of multiple gestations (all twins) was six with Org 32489 and three with urinary FSH. The implantation rate was 17% in the Org 32489 group and 13% in the urinary FSH group. None of the subjects had clinically relevant changes in biochemical variables and/or vital signs. Serum anti-FSH antibodies and anti-CHO cell-derived protein antibodies were not detected.

DISCUSSION

It was demonstrated here that treatment with either Org 32489 or urinary FSH was effective and safe in stimulating ovarian follicular development in infertile triptorelin-suppressed women undergoing IVF and embryo transfer. The number of oocytes retrieved as well as the pregnancy rates obtained seemed to be higher with Org 32489, but the between-group differences did not reach statistical significance. However, in a recently performed large multicentre study including 1000 first cycles in IVF with a similar design using buserelin as GnRH agonist, a significantly higher number of oocytes were retrieved after Org 32489 treatment (mean 10.8) as compared to urinary FSH (mean 9.0; 95% confidence interval and SE of treatment difference 1.2–2.6 and 0.4 respectively; Out *et al.*, 1995). In addition, in that study ongoing pregnancy rates were significantly higher after Org 32489 treatment when pregnancies resulting from frozen–thawed embryo replacements in subsequent natural cycles were included (25.7% versus 20.4%, $P = 0.05$). It might be that because of the small sample size of our study, which was not set up to detect small differences, the higher efficacy of Org 32489 as compared to urinary FSH was not apparent significantly.

The overall number of oocytes retrieved in the current study after Org 32489 treatment in triptorelin-suppressed women (mean ± SE 9.7 ± 1.3) compares well with other studies using Org 32489 but other GnRH agonists, with means ranging from nine to 11 (Devroey *et al.*, 1994; Out *et al.*, 1995).

Three cases of OHSS were reported as serious adverse events in the Org 32489 group (5.3%), including two ongoing pregnancies, whereas in the urinary FSH group the condition was not reported. The incidence of OHSS in our study was within the range that has been reported in other ovarian stimulation studies. In one subject in the urinary FSH group, abdominal pain was reported as a serious adverse event. Abdominal pain is a frequently reported adverse event during gonadotrophin treatment and is probably associated with ovarian stimulation which leads to some increase in the size of the ovary. Although Org 32489 differs slightly from natural FSH with respect to carbohydrate side-chain structure (Hård et al., 1990), and although the recombinant preparation contains minor amounts of proteins from the CHO cell line, antibody formation was not found in any of the Org 32489-treated subjects.

In summary, it can be concluded that in this prospective, randomized, assessor-blind, multicentre study, there was no statistically significant difference between Org 32489 (Puregon®) and urinary FSH (Metrodin®) in the outcome of ovarian stimulation in infertile triptorelin-suppressed women who were undergoing IVF and embryo transfer, as assessed by the number of oocytes retrieved. In addition, there were no apparent clinically relevant differences in the safety profile between Org 32489 and urinary FSH.

ACKNOWLEDGEMENTS

This study was financially supported by NV Organon, Oss, The Netherlands. The authors would like to thank the co-investigators I. Cedrin Durnerin (Bondy), C. Humeau, L. Lafont (Montpellier), B. Charbonnel, P. Barrière, F.X. Laurent (Nantes), I. Matheron (Paris), J. Belaisch-Allart, L. Nicolle (Sévres), and B. de Blank, A. Blum, P. Coudray, S. Driessen, F. Eikelboom, J. Geelen, P. Geurts, D. Rebrioux, I. van de Veerdonk (NV Organon).

REFERENCES

CPMP Working Party on Efficacy of Medicinal Products (1990) Good clinical practice for trials on medicinal products in the European Community. *Pharmacol. Toxicol.*, **67**, 361–372.

De Boer, W. and Mannaerts, B. (1990) Recombinant follicle stimulating hormone. II. Biochemical and biological characteristics. In Crommelin, D.J.A and Schellekens, H. (eds), *From Clone to Clinic, Developments in Biotherapy*. Kluwer Academic Publishers, Deventer, The Netherlands, pp. 253–259.

Devroey, P., Van Steirteghem, A., Mannaerts, B. and Coelingh Bennink, H. (1992a) Successful in-vitro fertilisation and embryo transfer after treatment with recombinant human FSH. *Lancet*, **339**, 1170–1171.

Devroey, P., Van Steirteghem, A., Mannaerts, B. and Coelingh Bennink, H. (1992b) First singleton term birth after ovarian superovulation with rhFSH. *Lancet*, **340**, 1108–1109.

Devroey, P., Mannaerts, B., Smitz, J., Coelingh Bennink, H. and Van Steirteghem, A. (1994) Clinical outcome of a pilot efficacy study on recombinant human follicle stimulating hormone (Org 32489) combined with various gonadotrophin-releasing hormone agonist regimens. *Hum. Reprod.*, **9**, 1064–1069.

Donderwinkel, P.F.J., Schoot, D.C., Coelingh Bennink, H.J.T. and Fauser, B.C.J.M. (1992) Pregnancy after induction of ovulation with recombinant human FSH in polycystic ovary syndrome. *Lancet*, **340**, 983–984.

Hård, K., Mekking, A., Damm, J.B.L., Kamerling, J.P., De Boer, W., Wijnands, R.A. and Vliegenthart, J.F.G. (1990) Isolation and structure determination of the intact sialylated N-linked carbohydrate chains of recombinant human follitropin expressed in Chinese hamster ovary cells. *Eur. J. Biochem.*, **193**, 263–271.

Keene, J.L., Matzuk, M.M., Otani, T., Fauser, B.C.J.M., Galway, A.B., Hsueh, A.J.W. and Boime, I. (1989) Expression of biologically active human follitropin in chinese hamster ovary cells. *J. Biol. Chem.*, **264**, 4769–4775.

Mannaerts, B., De Leeuw, R., Geelen, J., Van Ravenstein, A., Van Wezenbeek, P., Schuurs, A. and Kloosterboer, H. (1991) Comparative in vitro and in vivo studies on the biological properties of recombinant human follicle stimulating hormone. *Endocrinology*, **129**, 2623–2630.

Mannaerts, B., Shoham, Z., Schoot, D., Bouchard, P., Harlin, J., Fauser, B., Jacobs, H., Rombout, F. and Coelingh Bennink, H. (1993) Single-dose pharmacokinetics and pharmacodynamics of recombinant human follicle-stimulating hormone (Org 32489) in gonadotropin-deficient volunteers. *Fertil. Steril.*, **59**, 108–114.

Matikainen, T., De Leeuw, R., Mannaerts, B. and Huhtaniemi, I. (1994) Circulating bioactive and immuno-reactive recombinant human follicle stimulating hormone (Org 32489) after administration to gonadotropin-deficient subjects. *Fertil. Steril.*, **61**, 62–69.

Out, H.J., Mannaerts, B.M.J.L., Driessen, S.G.A.J. and Coelingh Bennink, H.J.T (for the European Puregon Collaborative IVF Study Group) (1995) A prospective, randomized, assessor-blind, multicentre study comparing recombinant and urinary follicle-stimulating hormone (Puregon vs Metrodin) in in-vitro fertilization. *Hum. Reprod.* **10**, 2534–2540.

Porcu, E., Fabbri, R., Dal Prato, L., Longhi, M., Seracchioli, R. and Flamigni, C. (1994) Comparison between depot and standard release triptoreline in in-vitro fertilization: pituitary sensitivity, luteal function, pregnancy outcome, and perinatal results. *Fertil. Steril.*, **62**, 126–132.

Schoot, D.C., Coelingh Bennink, H.J.T., Mannaerts, B.M.J.L., Lamberts, S.W.J., Bouchard, P and Fauser, B.C.J.M. (1992) Human recombinant follicle stimulating hormone induces growth of preovulatory follicles without concomitant increase in androgen and estrogen biosynthesis in a woman with isolated gonadotropin deficiency. *J. Clin. Endocrinol. Metab.*, **74**, 1471–1473

Schoot, D.C., Harlin, J., Shoham, Z., Mannaerts, B.M.J.L., Lahlou, N., Bouchard, P., Coelingh Bennink, H.J.T. and Fauser, B.C.J.M. (1994) Recombinant human follicle stimulating hormone and ovarian response in gonadotrophin-deficient women. *Hum. Reprod.*, **9**, 1237–1242.

Shoham, Z., Mannaerts, B., Insler, V. and Coelingh Bennink, H. (1993) Induction of follicular growth using recombinant human follicle stimulating hormone in two volunteer women with hypogonadotropic hypogonadism. *Fertil. Steril.*, **59**, 738–742.

Staessen, C., Camus, M., Khan, I., Smitz, J., Van Waesberghe, L., Wisanto, A., Devroey, P. and Van Steirteghem, A.C. (1989) An 18-month survey of infertility treatment by in vitro fertilization, gamete and zygote intrafallopian transfer, and replacement of frozen-thawed embryos. *J. In Vitro Fertil. Embryo Transfer*, **6**, 22–29.

Van Dessel, H.J.H.M., Donderwinkel, P.F.J., Coelingh Bennink, H.J.T. and Fauser, B.C.J.M. (1994) First established pregnancy and birth after induction of ovulation with recombinant human follicle stimulating hormone in polycystic ovary syndrome. *Hum. Reprod.*, **9**, 55–56.

Van Wezenbeek, P., Draaijer, J., Van Meel, F. and Olijve, W. (1990) Recombinant follicle stimulating hormone. I. Construction, selection and characterization of a cell line. In Crommelin, D.J.A. and Schellekens, H. (eds), *From Clone to Clinic, Developments in Biotherapy*. Kluwer Academic Publishers, Deventer, The Netherlands, pp. 245–251.

Whitehead, A. and Whitehead, J. (1991) A general parametric approach to the meta-analysis of randomized clinical trials. *Statist. Med.*, **10**, 1665–1667.

Received June 1, 1995; accepted September 1, 1995

Correspondence: H.J. Out, NV Organon, PO Box 20, BH 5340 Oss, The Netherlands

13

A prospective, randomized, assessor-blind, multicentre study comparing recombinant and urinary follicle stimulating hormone (Puregon versus Metrodin) in in-vitro fertilization

H.J. Out*, B.M.J.L. Mannaerts*, S.G.A.J. Driessen[†] and H.J.T. Coelingh Bennink*

*Section Reproductive Medicine and [†]Biometrics, Medical Research and Development Unit, NV Organon, PO Box 20, 5340 BH Oss, The Netherlands

ABSTRACT

Urinary follicle stimulating hormone (FSH) is being used for the treatment of human infertility. Recently, FSH manufactured by means of recombinant DNA technology with a much higher purity (>99%) has become available. A prospective, randomized, assessor-blind, multicentre (n = 18) study was conducted in infertile women undergoing in-vitro fertilization comparing recombinant FSH (Org 32489, Puregon®) and urinary FSH (Metrodin®). Eligible subjects were randomized (recombinant versus urinary FSH = 3:2) and pretreated with buserelin for pituitary suppression. FSH was given until three or more follicles with a diameter of at least 17 mm were seen. After oocyte retrieval, fertilization routines were applied according to local procedures. No more than three embryos were replaced. In all, 585 subjects received recombinant FSH and 396 urinary FSH. Significantly more oocytes were retrieved after recombinant FSH treatment (mean adjusted for centre 10.84 versus 8.95, $P < 0.0001$). Ongoing pregnancy rates per attempt and transfer in the recombinant FSH group were 22.17 and 25.97% respectively, and in the urinary FSH group, 18.22 and 22.02% respectively (not significant). Ongoing pregnancy rates including pregnancies resulting from frozen-thawed embryo cycles were 25.7% for recombinant and 20.4% for urinary FSH ($P = 0.05$). Compared to urinary FSH, the total

This paper was first published in *Human Reproduction*, **10** (10) 2534–2540 (1995). Copyright 1995 Oxford University Press, reproduced with permission *dose of FSH was significantly lower with recombinant FSH (2138 versus 2385 IU, P < 0.0001) in a significantly shorter treatment period (10.7 versus 11.3 days, P < 0.0001). No clinically relevant differences between recombinant and urinary FSH were seen with respect to safety variables. It is concluded that recombinant FSH (Puregon) is more effective than urinary FSH in inducing multifollicular development and achieving an ongoing pregnancy.*

INTRODUCTION

For >30 years, human menopausal gonadotrophins (HMG) have been applied in the treatment of human infertility. Clinical applications include ovulation induction in clomiphene-resistant anovulatory women and ovarian stimulation in assisted reproduction techniques, e.g. in-vitro fertilisation (IVF) (Breckwoldt and Zahradnik, 1991). Most HMG preparations contain either equal amounts of follicle stimulating hormone (FSH) and luteinizing hormone (LH) activity (FSH/LH ratio = 1) or mainly FSH activity with minor amounts of LH activity (urofollitrophin, FSH/LH ratio ≥60). The production of these hormones depends on the collection of huge amounts of urine. The use of urine sources implies limited product consistency and purity (1–5%).

Recently, FSH has been manufactured by means of recombinant DNA technology using a Chinese hamster ovary (CHO) cell line transfected with the genes encoding human FSH (Van Wezenbeek *et al.*, 1990). The final product (Org 32489, Puregon®) is purified up to 99% purity, does not contain any LH activity and is very similar to natural FSH (Hård *et al.*, 1990), although small differences in oligosaccharide moieties and isohormone composition are present.

Clinical experiences with recombinant FSH indicate the potential of the compound to induce follicular growth, and pregnancy can be achieved (Devroey *et al.*, 1994). In this paper, a multicentre trial is described evaluating the efficacy and safety of recombinant FSH to achieve ovarian stimulation in infertile women undergoing IVF, in comparison with urinary FSH.

MATERIALS AND METHODS

Patients

Between March 1992 and August 1993, infertile female subjects were recruited at 18 different IVF centres throughout Europe (see Acknowledgements section). The aim was to include 1000 patients. Inclusion criteria were as follows: patients had to be 18–39 years of age at the time of screening; have a cause of infertility which was potentially solvable by IVF; a maximum of three previous IVF or other assisted reproduction attempts in which oocytes were collected at least once; normal ovulatory cycles with a mean length of between 24 and 35 days and an intra-individual variation of plus or minus 3 days (but never outside the 24–35 days range); good physical and mental health; and a body weight 80–130% of the ideal body weight (adapted from the Metropolitan Life Insurance Company Tables).

Exclusion criteria were: infertility caused by endocrine abnormalities such as hyperprolactinaemia, polycystic ovary syndrome, and absence of ovarian function; male infertility as defined by $<10 \times 10^6$ spermatozoa/ml and/or <40% normal morphology and/or <40% normal motility; any ovarian and/or abdominal abnormality that would interfere with adequate ultrasound investigation; hypertension (sitting diastolic blood pressure >90 mmHg and/or systolic blood pressure >150 mmHg); chronic cardiovascular, hepatic, renal, or pulmonary disease; a history of (within 12 months) or current abuse of alcohol or drugs; administration of non-registered investigational drugs within 3 months prior to screening. When all criteria were met, the subject was considered to be eligible. The study was approved by the Ethics Committee of each local hospital. All subjects gave written informed consent. This investigation was performed according to the Declaration of Helsinki and the European Community note on Good Clinical Practice for trials on medicinal products in the European Community (CPMP Working Party on Efficacy of Medicinal Products, 1990).

Study design

This was a randomized, assessor-blind, prospective, multicentre study comparing recombinant human FSH (Org 32489, Puregon®, NV Organon, Oss, The Netherlands, batch numbers CP 091134 and 091077) and urinary FSH (urofollitropin, Metrodin®, Ares-Serono, Switzerland, batch numbers CP 092139, 093057, 092047, 091163). The objective of the study was to assess the efficacy and safety of recombinant FSH in relation to urinary FSH for the induction of ovarian stimulation in infertile pituitary-suppressed subjects undergoing IVF. Eligible subjects were randomized by receiving a subject number from a randomization list corresponding with patient boxes in which the medication was kept. The randomization procedure included a ratio between recombinant and urinary FSH of 3:2. All centres followed an identical clinical protocol and used standardized case report forms.

Pituitary down-regulation started on the first day of the menstruation by means of intranasal buserelin (Suprecur®, Hoechst, Germany). The initial dose was $4 \times 150\,\mu g$ daily. When suppression was not achieved (serum oestradiol >200 pmol/l) after 14 days, the dose was doubled ($4 \times 300\,\mu g$ daily). The buserelin intake was sustained throughout the FSH treatment. The FSH dose for the first 4 days was 150 or 225 IU (two or three ampoules i.m.). Afterwards, the dose was adjusted according to follicular development as assessed by ultrasound scanning. Since, for technical reasons, recombinant FSH was supplied in vials and urinary FSH in ampoules, a double-blind design was not feasible. Instead, an assessor-blind design was chosen in which preparation and administration of the medication was done by a study co-ordinator who took no part in any decision concerning the FSH dose during treatment. When at least three follicles ≥17 mm were present, 10 000 IU of human chorionic gonadotrophin (HCG, Pregnyl®, NV Organon, The Netherlands) was given i.m. to induce ovulation. Oocyte retrieval, fertilization procedures and embryo transfer were done according to the local standards. A maximum of three embryos was transferred. Luteal support was given during at least 2 weeks and included minimally three injections of 1500 IU HCG or at least 50 mg of progesterone daily i.m. or 400 mg progesterone daily intravaginally.

End-points

The primary outcome variables were the number of oocytes retrieved, and ongoing pregnancy rate per attempt and transfer as assessed by ultrasound scanning at least 12 weeks following embryo transfer.

Secondary variables included number of follicles ≥15 mm and ≥17 mm on the day of HCG administration, length of FSH treatment, total dose, serum concentrations of FSH and oestradiol on the day of administering HCG, number of mature oocytes recovered, number of high quality embryos, implantation rate, clinical pregnancy rates per attempt and transfer. Implantation rate was defined as the number of vital fetuses as assessed by ultrasound at least 12 weeks after embryo transfer, divided by the number of embryos transferred for each subject. The definition of a clinical pregnancy included miscarriages with or without proof of a vital fetus.

Fertilization and cleavage rates are not reported due to the heterogeneity in IVF routines across the centres.

The main safety parameters were the incidence of ovarian hyperstimulation syndrome (OHSS) and the development of anti-FSH antibodies and anti-CHO cell-derived protein antibodies. Also, common laboratory parameters were compared before and after treatment. These parameters included routine blood biochemistry as sodium, potassium, chloride, bicarbonate, phosphorus, calcium, glucose, urea, creatinine, alkaline phosphatase, alanine amino transferase, aspartase amino transferase, lactic dehydrogenase, total bilirubin, total protein, albumin; haematology parameters included haemoglobin, haematocrit, erythrocytes, leukocytes plus differentiation; urinalysis included quantitative estimation of pH and qualitative estimations of protein, acetone, glucose, and haemoglobin.

Assessments

At screening, the medical history was obtained and a physical examination was performed. Routine blood biochemistry, haematology and urinalysis were done and the following endocrinological parameters were measured: serum oestradiol, FSH, LH, progesterone, testosterone, prolactin, and dehydroepiandrosterone sulphate. An ultrasound scan was done to exclude ovarian abnormalities. Sperm analysis of the partner took place and was repeated at the time of fertilization.

Serum oestradiol concentrations were measured to ensure optimal pituitary suppression prior to the first FSH injection. Serum FSH, LH, oestradiol and progesterone were measured on the first day of FSH treatment and on the day of HCG administration. In between, assessments of serum oestradiol and LH were done on a regular basis. Frequent ultrasound scans were made to monitor follicular growth.

Spare serum samples for the determination of anti-FSH and anti-CHO-cell derived protein antibodies were taken before and after treatment. Routine blood biochemistry, haematology and urinalysis were repeated as soon as possible after FSH treatment had ended.

Classification of oocytes as either mature or immature and embryos as type 1, 2, 3, or 4 was done according to previously published criteria (Staessen *et al.*, 1989). Type 1 and 2 were considered to be high quality embryos.

Assays

Antibody assay

Blood samples processed to serum taken before and after FSH treatment were sent to NV Organon, The Netherlands for central determination of anti-FSH and anti-CHO cell-derived protein antibodies.

Anti-FSH antibodies The presence of specific antibodies against human FSH was assessed by a semi-quantitative radioimmunoassay in duplicate. In short, ^{125}I-labelled recombinant FSH was allowed to react with antibodies present in the sample. The immune-complexes formed were subsequently precipitated with polyethylene glycol (PEG 8000). After removal of the supernatant, bound radioactivity in the pellet was quantified. A calibration curve with human anti-FSH antibodies that would allow quantitative determination of the serum anti-FSH antibody concentration could not be established, since there is no representative standard human anti-FSH antibody preparation available. Therefore, all values were expressed as percentage of the total amount of tracer added in the assay and were corrected for the non-specific binding. Clinically relevant antibody titres were defined as those yielding a binding percentage of >25%.

Anti-CHO cell-derived protein antibodies The occurrence of antibodies against proteins from the CHO cell line was assessed by a semi-quantitative enzyme-immunoassay. In short, CHO cell-derived proteins were coated to the wall of 96-well microtitre plates. Antibodies in the sample were allowed to bind to the solid-phase-coated CHO cell-derived proteins, where they were then detected with a horseradish peroxidase coupled second antibody [goat antihuman immunoglobulin (IgG)]. The end product of the enzyme reaction was quantified spectrophotometrically at 450 nm, corrected for the optical density at 690 nm. Each analytical run included a series of six concentrations in human serum of the IgG fraction of a rabbit polyclonal antiserum against CHO cell-derived proteins as positive control. The CHO cell-derived proteins used to obtain this antiserum and the CHO cell-derived proteins applied in the assay were purified from the culture supernatant of a mock-transfected CHO cell line.

Other assays

Sperm analysis and measurement of blood biochemistry, haematology, urinalysis and endocrinological parameters were done at the local hospital according to local standards. Follicular size was measured with local ultrasound equipment and a vaginal probe.

Sample size

Power calculations were performed in order to assess the magnitude of treatment effects capable of detection in this large study, and were based on efficacy data of 1000 subjects, assuming that at least 850 subjects had an oocyte retrieval and embryo transfer (Dupont and Plummer, 1990). When testing at the customary 5% significance level (two-sided), and assuming an SD of 6, a difference of 1.2 oocytes in the two treatment groups would have been detected statistically with a probability of 80%. With respect to dichotomous variables such as pregnancy, by assuming a pregnancy rate of 15% per attempt and 18% per transfer for one treatment group, a value per attempt (and transfer) as small as 9% (11%) or as large as 22% (26%) for the second group would have been detected statistically with an 80% probability, using a two-sided χ^2 test, again at the 5% significance level. Therefore, the size of the study ensured that fairly modest treatment effects would have been detected with a high probability.

Statistical analysis

For ordinal data a general parametric approach (Whitehead and Whitehead, 1991) of combining individual centre results was applied and used for communication of results and eventual analysis. For binary data (pregnancy outcome) the Mantel–Haenszel test statistic extended for multiple centres was used. In both cases the combination of centre results was expressed as means adjusted for centre and approximate confidence intervals (CI) were calculated based on the normal distribution.

All analyses were done on an intent-to-treat basis, including all subjects who received at least one ampoule of FSH. The main advantages of this rule were that more patients were available for final analysis of efficacy and that it more closely reflected how physicians evaluate a therapeutic agent in the clinical setting, outside an experimental control.

RESULTS

Patients

A total of 1027 subjects (recombinant FSH: n = 615, urinary FSH: n = 412) was randomized, 1007 (recombinant FSH: n = 602, urinary FSH: n = 405) started buserelin pretreatment and 981 (recombinant FSH: n = 585, urinary FSH: n = 396) started FSH treatment. The number of subjects treated with FSH per centre was 10–146 (mean 54.5).

Both treatment groups were comparable in demographic and infertility characteristics (Table 1). The main cause of infertility was tubal disease (64.4 and 64.1% for recombinant versus urinary FSH respectively).

Table 1 Demographic and infertility characteristics

Characteristic	Recombinant FSH (n = 585)	Urinary FSH (n = 396)
Mean age (years)	32.2	32.3
Mean weight (kg)	61.3	61.2
Mean height (cm)	164.4	164.3
Number (%) of subjects with cause of infertility		
tubal disease	377 (64.4)	254 (64.1)
endometriosis	45 (7.7)	30 (7.6)
tubal disease + endometriosis	23 (3.9)	15 (3.8)
unknown	117 (20.0)	79 (19.9)
other	23 (3.9)	18 (4.5)
Mean duration of infertility (years)	6.3	6.1
Number (%) of subjects with primary infertility	259 (44.3)	174 (43.9)
Number (%) of subjects with secondary infertility	326 (55.7)	222 (56.1)

The mean duration of infertility for recombinant and urinary FSH was 6.3 and 6.1 years respectively.

Primary efficacy parameters

The results of the main efficacy parameters are given in Table 2. In the recombinant FSH group, a mean number (adjusted for centre) of 10.84 oocytes was recovered, compared to 8.95 in the urinary FSH group. The difference of 1.89 was highly significant ($P < 0.0001$; 95% CI 1.2–2.6). The mean number of oocytes recovered across the centres ranged from 7.2 to 16.4 for recombinant FSH and from 4.0 to 12.8 for urinary FSH, the differences varying from 0.62 to 5.50 oocytes. In all centres, more oocytes were retrieved after recombinant FSH treatment (Figure 1).

Ongoing pregnancy rates per attempt and transfer and adjusted for centre were 22.17 and 25.97% respectively for the recombinant FSH group, and 18.22 and 22.02% respectively, in the urinary FSH group. Until August 1994, 117 and 73 subjects in the recombinant and urinary FSH group respectively, subsequently underwent a natural cycle during which frozen-thawed embryos were replaced, resulting in 17 ongoing pregnancies in the recombinant FSH group and five in the urinary FSH group. A second 'frozen embryo' cycle was done in 26 and 15 women,

Table 2 Results on main parameters

Parameter	Mean adjusted for centre		Recombinant minus urinary FSH		
	Recombinant FSH	Urinary FSH	Difference	SE	95% CI
No. of oocytes recovered	10.84	8.95	1.89	0.37	1.2–2.6 ($P < 0.0001$)
Ongoing pregnancy rate per attempt (%)	22.17	18.22	3.95	2.59	–1.1–9.0 NS
Ongoing pregnancy rate per transfer (%)	25.97	22.02	3.95	3.01	–1.9–9.8 NS

CI = confidence interval.
NS = not significant.

which resulted in seven additional pregnancies: five in the recombinant and two in the urinary FSH group. Eight women had a third frozen embryo cycle and two subjects a fourth, which did not result in ongoing pregnancies. The mean number of embryos transferred in the frozen embryo cycles was 2.1 for both groups. In total, 22 additional pregnancies were obtained in the recombinant FSH group, and seven in the urinary FSH group, resulting in cumulative ongoing pregnancy rates (adjusted for centre) of 25.7 and 20.4% in favour of recombinant FSH (P = 0.05).

Secondary efficacy parameters

Results of the secondary parameters are given in Table 3. On the day of HCG, significantly more follicles ≥15 mm were seen in the recombinant FSH group (n = 7.49, mean adjusted for centre), compared to the urinary FSH group (n = 6.67, P = 0.0002, 95% CI of difference: 0.4–1.2). Figure 2 demonstrates that development of large (≥15 mm) follicles began to diverge between the groups after 5–6 days of FSH treatment. This higher number of follicles was associated with a significantly increased maximum serum oestradiol in the recombinant FSH group (mean adjusted for centre 6084 versus 5179 pmol/l, P < 0.0001). On the day of HCG, FSH concentrations were significantly higher in the urinary FSH group (12.1 versus 11.5 IU/l, P = 0.03). A significantly lower total dose of recombinant FSH (mean adjusted for centre 2138 versus 2385 IU, P < 0.0001) were needed in an also significantly shorter

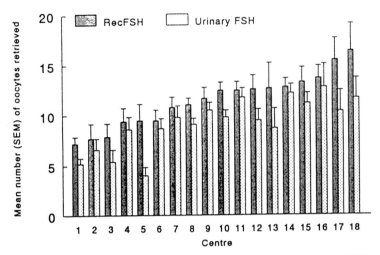

Figure 1 Mean (±SEM) number of oocytes retrieved per centre. FSH = follicle stimulating hormone. Rec = recombinant

treatment period (10.7 versus 11.3 days, P < 0.0001) compared to the urinary FSH group. There was no linear relationship between the number of ampoules administered and number of oocytes collected.

Mean LH concentrations after down-regulation before start of the FSH treatment were 1.6 and 1.7 IU/l, and on the day of HCG administration 1.2 and 1.3 IU/l in the recombinant and urinary FSH groups respectively.

After oocyte retrieval, more mature oocytes (difference 1.8, P < 0.0001; 95% CI 1.1–2.4) were recovered and more high quality embryos (difference 0.5, P = 0.003; 95% CI 0.2–0.8) were obtained in the recombinant FSH group.

No significant differences between recombinant and urinary FSH were seen in the number of follicles ≥17 mm on the day of HCG, the implantation rate and the clinical pregnancy rates per attempt and transfer (see Table 3).

The mean number of oocytes with two pronuclei was 6.8 and 5.6 in the recombinant and urinary FSH groups respectively, as assessed 12–18 h after incubation with semen. Oocytes with three or more pronuclei were seen in 208 subjects (38.2%) in the recombinant FSH group, compared to 117 (32.4%) in the urinary FSH group. A mean number of 2.58 and 1.81 embryos were frozen in the recombinant and urinary FSH groups respectively.

Table 3 Results on secondary parameters

Parameter	Mean adjusted for centre			Recombinant minus urinary FSH		
	Recombinant FSH	Urinary FSH	Difference	SE	95% CI	
No. of follicles ≥15 mm on day of HCG	7.49	6.67	0.81	0.22	0.41–1.2 ($P = 0.0002$)	
No. of follicles ≥17 mm on day of HCG	4.61	4.38	0.23	0.14	−0.0–0.5 NS	
Maximum serum oestradiol (pmol/l)	6084	5179	905	210	494–1317 ($P < 0.0001$)	
Serum FSH on day of HCG (IU/l)	11.5	12.1	−0.6	0.26	−1.1 to −0.1 ($P = 0.03$)	
Total no. of ampoules used	28.5	31.8	−3.3	0.62	−4.5 to −2.1 ($P < 0.0001$)	
Treatment length (days)	10.7	11.3	−0.6	0.13	−0.9 to −0.3 ($P < 0.0001$)	
No. of mature oocytes recovered	8.55	6.76	1.79	0.33	1.1–2.4 ($P < 0.0001$)	
No. of high quality embryos	3.11	2.61	0.50	0.17	0.2–0.8 ($P = 0.003$)	
Implantation rate (%)	0.11	0.09	0.01	0.02	−0.02–0.05 NS	
Clinical pregnancy rate (%) per attempt	29.29	25.30	3.99	2.88	−1.6–9.6 NS	
Clinical pregnancy rate (%) per transfer	34.30	30.46	3.84	3.31	−2.6–10.3 NS	

CI = confidence interval; NS = not significant; HCG = human chorionic gonadotrophin; FSH = follicle stimulating hormone.

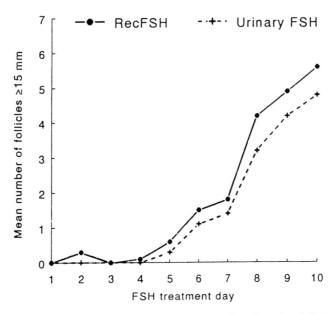

Figure 2 Mean number of follicles ≥15 mm related to the follicle stimulating hormone (FSH) treatment day. Rec = recombinant

Cycle cancellations

In all, 152 patients started FSH treatment but did not have an embryo transfer (recombinant FSH: n = 85, 14.5%; urinary FSH: n = 67, 16.9%; not significantly different). Low ovarian response was reported in 27 subjects in the recombinant FSH group (4.6%) and in 30 in the urinary FSH group (7.6%). The risk of OHSS was the reason for cancellation in 12 recombinant FSH-treated subjects (2.1%) and six urinary FSH-treated subjects (1.5%). Unsuccessful fertilization was the reason for premature discontinuation in 29 subjects (5.0%) in the recombinant FSH group, compared to 16 (4.0%) in the urinary FSH group.

Safety

OHSS leading to hospitalization was seen in 19 out of 585 recombinant FSH-treated subjects (3.2%) compared with eight out of 396 urinary FSH-treated subjects (2.0%, not significantly different). In 545 recombinant FSH-treated and 353 urinary FSH-treated subjects spare serum samples could be assessed for the presence of anti-FSH and anti-CHO cell-derived protein antibodies. No significant rises of serum antibody concentrations were found. Clinically relevant changes from base line of routine blood biochemistry, haematology and urinalysis were not detected.

DISCUSSION

To our knowledge, this is the largest prospective, randomized clinical trial ever performed in IVF. In total, 585 subjects received recombinant FSH (Puregon®) and 396 urinary FSH (Metrodin®) for ovarian stimulation. The aim of stimulation was to increase the number of oocytes for assisted reproduction. Therefore, the number of oocytes retrieved was chosen as one of the main efficacy parameters in this study. Ovarian stimulation was continued until there was evidence of adequate multiple follicular development (at least three follicles ≥17 mm in diameter). The fact that the treatment groups did not differ significantly with respect to the number of follicles ≥17 mm on the day of HCG indicated that the stimulation procedures were carried out in a similar way. However, a significantly higher number of oocytes was retrieved in the recombinant FSH group. Despite the large well-known differences between centres in overall number of oocytes retrieved, this finding was consistently in favour of recombinant FSH throughout all centres (Figure 1). Accordingly, a larger cohort of follicles was recruited in these subjects, as illustrated by the significantly higher number of follicles ≥15 mm in the recombinant FSH group seen on the last ultrasound before oocyte retrieval. The significantly higher maximum serum oestradiol concentration in the recombinant FSH group is most likely a reflection of this larger number of follicles. Interestingly, overall concentrations of immunoreactive FSH on the day of HCG were slightly but significantly lower in the recombinant FSH group, even though different types of FSH assays were applied which increased the overall variability. This might be related to the significantly lower amount of recombinant FSH administered and the significantly shorter treatment period in this group. It also illustrates that FSH concentrations based on immunoassay measurements have only limited value in assessing the true potency, since they only reflect the number of circulating FSH molecules but not their actual biological activity.

According to pharmacopeial requirements (Council of Europe, 1986), the FSH activity of a batch is calibrated in the in-vivo Steelman–Pohley rat assay, against an International Standard Preparation (Steelman and Pohley, 1953). This rat model is apparently not valid to predict clinical activity in the human, given the differences we found using nominally equal preparations with the same declared content, namely 75 IU in-vivo bioactivity per ampoule.

Possible factors which might explain the higher potency of recombinant FSH compared to urinary FSH include subtle differences at the level of the oligosaccharide moieties of the molecules, differences in isohormone composition (Matikainen *et al.*, 1994), or the proteinaceous contaminants in the urinary product inhibiting FSH action and the pharmaceutical formulation. Further research is needed to elucidate the influence of these factors on the clinical efficacy of gonadotrophin preparations. Not all recombinant FSH products give identical results with IVF, or are superior to urinary FSH (recombinant human FSH study group, 1995). In fact, in that study oestradiol levels at the day of HCG administration were significantly lower in the recombinant FSH group. This surely suggests that differences between various recombinant FSH preparations exist.

With respect to the other main efficacy parameter, ongoing pregnancy rate, no statistically significant difference between the recombinant and urinary FSH groups was found. This is to be expected since the significant treatment differences in favour of recombinant FSH, such as the higher number of oocytes retrieved and the larger number of high quality embryos, are basically nullified since both groups 'restarted' treatment at an equal position at the moment of transfer of a fixed maximum number of embryos. In both treatment groups a mean of 2.4 embryos were replaced. However, differences in ongoing pregnancy rates including 'frozen embryo' cycles reached statistical significance in favour of recombinant FSH ($P = 0.05$). This might be due to the availability of better quality embryos after recombinant FSH treatment, next to the obvious reason that merely the presence of more embryos ultimately will lead to more pregnancies.

The most important side-effect of gonadotrophin treatment in ovarian stimulation is the occurrence of OHSS. This possibly life-threatening condition is characterized in its most serious forms by ascites, haemoconcentration, coagulation and electrolyte disorders and extreme ovarian enlargement (Rizk and Smitz, 1992). Despite the higher number of follicles recruited and the increased serum oestradiol concentration on the day of HCG administration, which are both risk factors for the development of the syndrome, its incidence was not statistically significantly higher after recombinant FSH treatment. However, the incidence of severe hyperstimulation requiring hospitalization is so low that the power of the study would be insufficient to detect a significant difference of 2%. Therefore, given the higher potency of recombinant FSH, careful monitoring to prevent the occurrence of this syndrome is essential.

Recombinant and natural FSH differ slightly at the level of carbohydrate moieties (Hård *et al.*, 1990) and potentially, minute amounts of host cell-originating contaminations might be present in the recombinant preparation. To investigate the immunogenic characteristics, and to rule out any risk, antibody development against FSH and CHO cell-derived proteins was assayed. Antibody formation was not seen in any of the recombinant FSH-treated patients.

In conclusion, this study has demonstrated that recombinant FSH (Puregon®) is more efficacious than urinary FSH (Metrodin®) as assessed by the number of oocytes retrieved. Pregnancy rates including frozen embryo cycles were significantly higher after recombinant FSH treatment. Recombinant and urinary FSH are equally safe.

ACKNOWLEDGEMENTS

The European Puregon® collaborative IVF study group consists of:

Belgium: Centre for Reproductive Medicine, Academic Hospital Free University, Brussels; P. Devroey, A. van Steirteghem, J. Smitz.

Denmark: Rikshospitalet, Department of Gynaecology, Fertility Clinic, Copenhagen; P. Hornnes.

Finland: Department of Obstetrics and Gynaecology, Helsinki University Central Hospital, Helsinki; A. Tiitinen, N. Simberg, M. Tulppala, M.T. Seppälä.

Germany: Universitäts-Frauenklinik, Bonn; K. Diedrich, C. Diedrich. Universitäts-Frauenklinik, Erlangen; L. Wildt, E. Siebzehnrübl, B. Munzer.

Greece: Infertility and IVF Centre 'Geniki Cliniki', Thessaloniki; B.C. Tarlatzis, J. Bontis, S. Lagos, H. Bili, D. Bakratsa, S. Mantalenakis.

Ireland: Human Assisted Reproduction Ireland, RCSI Academic Department of Obstetrics and Gynaecology, Rotunda Hospital, Dublin; R.K. Harrison, U. Kondaveeti, B. Hennelly, A. Gordon, L. Drudy, E. Cottell, A. MacMahon.

Israel: Department of Obstetrics and Gynaecology, Kaplan Hospital, Rehovoth; Z. Shoham, A. Barash, P. Golan, I. Segal, L. Sindel, V. Insler.

Norway: Kvinnekliniken Rikshopitalet, Oslo; T. Åbyholm, T. Tanbo, L. Henriksen. Kvinneklinikken Regionsykehuset i Trondheim, Trondheim; J. Kahn, A. Sunde, L. Reinertsen.

Spain: Servicio de Reprodución Humana, Instituto Dexeus, Barcelona; R Barri, R Cabrero, M. Torello.

Sweden: Kvinnokliniken, Sahigrenska sjukhuset, Göteborg; L. Hamberger, L. Nilsson, C. Bergh, A. Strandell, B. Josefsson. Department of Obstetrics and Gynaecology, University of Lund, Malmö; N.O. Sjöberg, L. Hägglund, F. Ploman.

UK: Department of Obstetrics and Gynaecology, Guy's Hospital, London; R.G. Forman, S.A. Adeaga. Regional IVF Unit, St Mary's Hospital, Manchester; B. Lieberman, P. Buck, P. Matson, F. Hamer, A. Ratcliffe, J. Bent, G. Horne. Department of Obstetrics and Gynaecology, University of Wales College of Medicine, Cardiff; R.W. Shaw, S. Vine. The Assisted Conception Unit, Royal Infirmary of Edinburgh, Edinburgh; C.P. West, H. Hillier. Hammersmith Royal Postgraduate Medical School, Institute of Obstetrics and Gynaecology, London and IVF Clinic, Royal Masonic Hospital, London; R.M.L. Winston, N. Reddy, G. Atkinson, A. Huodono.

NV Organon, Oss, The Netherlands: B. de Blank, W. de Boer, H. Coelingh Bennink, S. Driessen, E Eikelboom, J. Geelen, R Janssen, H. Joosten, R. de Leeuw, B. Mannaerts, F. van Meel, A. de Meere, F. Metsers, J. Mulders, H.J. Out, R. Paulussen, F. Rombout, A. Skrabanja, I. van de Veerdonk, R. Verbeeten, J. Verhoeven, and many others.

REFERENCES

Breckwoldt, M. and Zahradnik, H.P. (1991) Induction of ovulation with human gonadotropins. In Coelingh Bennink, H.J.T., Vemer, H.M., and Van Keep, P.A. (eds), *Chronic Hyperandrogenic Anovulation*. Parthenon Publishing, Carnforth.

Council of Europe (1986) *European Pharmacopoeia*, 2nd edn, pp. 508-1 to 508-4.

CPMP Working Party on Efficacy of Medicinal Products (1990) Good clinical practice for trials on medicinal products in the European Community. *Pharmacol. Toxicol.*, **67**, 361–372.

Devroey, P., Mannaerts, B., Smitz, J., Coelingh Bennink, H. and Van Steirteghem, A. (1994) Clinical outcome of a pilot efficacy study on recombinant human follicle-stimulating hormone (Org 32489) combined with various gonadotrophin-releasing hormone agonist regimens. *Hum. Reprod.*, **9**, 1064–1069.

Dupont, W.D. and Plummer, W.D. (1990) Power and sample size calculations, a review and computer program. *Controlled Clin. Trials,* **11**, 116–128.

Hård, K., Mekking, A., Damm, J.B.L., Kamerling, J.R., De Boer, W., Wijnands, R.A. and Vliegenthart, J.F.G. (1990) Isolation and structure determination of the intact sialylated N-linked carbohydrate chains of recombinant human follitropin (hFSH) expressed in Chinese Hamster ovary cells. *Eur. J. Biochem.*, **193**, 263–271.

Matikainen, T., De Leeuw, R., Mannaerts, B. and Huhtaniemi, I. (1994) Circulating bioactive and immunoreactive recombinant human follicle-stimulating hormone (Org 32489) after administration to gonadotropin-deficient subjects. *Fertil. Steril.*, **61**, 62–69.

Recombinant human FSH study group (1995) Clinical assessment of recombinant human follicle-stimulating hormone in stimulating ovarian follicular development before in-vitro fertilization. *Fertil. Steril.*, **63**, 77–86.

Rizk, B. and Smitz, I. (1992) Ovarian hyperstimulation syndrome after superovulation using GnRH agonists for IVF and related procedures. *Hum. Reprod.*, **7**, 320–327.

Staessen, C., Camus, M., Khan, I., Smitz, I., Van Waesberghe, L., Wisanto, A., Devroey, P. and Van Steirteghem, A.C. (1989) An 18-month survey of infertility treatment by in vitro fertilization, gamete and zygote intrafallopian transfer, and replacement of frozen-thawed embryos. *J. In Vitro Fertil. Embryo Transfer*, **6**, 22–29.

Steelman, S.L. and Pohley, F. (1953) Assay of the follicle stimulating hormone based on the augmentation with human chorionic gonadotropin. *Endocrinology*, **53**, 604–616.

Van Wezenbeek, P., Draaijer, J., Van Meel, F. and Olijve, W. (1990) Recombinant follicle stimulating hormone. I. Construction, selection and characterization of a cell line. In Crommelin, D.J.A. and Schellekens, H. (eds), *From Clone to Clinic, Developments in Biotherapy*. Kluwer Academic Publications, pp. 245–251.

Whitehead, A. and Whitehead, J. (1991) A general parametric approach to the meta-analysis of randomised clinical trials. *Stat. Med.*, **10**, 1665–1677.

Received October 4, 1994; accepted July 20, 1995

Correspondence: H.J.T. Coelingh Bennink, Section Reproductive Medicine, NV Organon, PO Box 20, 5340 BH Oss, The Netherlands

Index

absorption rate 45, 94–95
  sex differences 86, 94–95
androstenedione
  production 4, 51, 54, 62, 126
  serum levels 120–121, 125
aromatase activity 4, 13–18, 81
  effects of hCG supplementation 4, 13, 18
  effects of recombinant versus natural FSH 15–16
atresia, follicular 49, 54–63

birth
  efficacy study 100, 108
  first case report 69–73
  with polycystic ovary syndrome 131–134
body weight, serum FSH levels and 86, 92–93, 95

Chinese hamster ovary (CHO) cell line 5
chromatofocusing 39–40, 45
cumulus–corona–oocyte complexes 100, 107–108

dominant follicles 31–32

efficacy
  case study 99–110
  parameters
    primary 151, 164–165
    secondary 151, 165–167
  recombinant versus natural FSH 143–154, 157–171
embryo transfer 100, 107–108
  recombinant versus natural FSH 157, 164–165
  see also in vitro fertilization
endometrial proliferation 49–50, 56–58, 63, 64
estradiol
  intraovarian production 49–50, 53–54, 62
  granulosa cell responses 23, 26–32
  LH role 75–81
  plasma levels 4, 13–16, 53–54, 62
    case studies 80, 107, 109, 120–124, 126
    first established pregnancy 70–72
    hCG supplementation effects 4, 13–16
    recombinant versus natural FSH 151–152, 165, 169–170
  role in follicular development 126–127
estrogen synthesis
  LH importance 75–81
  two-cell two-gonadotropin theory 4–5, 18
  see also estradiol

follicle stimulating hormone (FSH)
  comparison with recFSH 3–19, 143–154, 157–171
  bioactivity following single injection 35–46
  effects on granulosa cells 26–28
  efficacy 143–154, 157–171
  immunoreactivity following single injection 35–46
  in vitro bioassay studies 3, 7–11
  in vitro neutralization of bioactivity 10, 13
  receptor displacement studies 3, 7, 10, 12, 17
  safety 143–154
  immunoassay 6
  mechanism of action 4
  role in follicular development 18, 24, 49–64
  see also recombinant FSH
  serum levels 75, 79–80
    body weight and 86, 92–93
    efficacy study 106–107
    first established pregnancy 70–71
    following multiple-dose administration 115–116, 120–125

175

recombinant versus natural FSH
152, 165–166
single-dose pharmacokinetics
35–46, 86, 90–92
follicles
  atresic 54–63
  dominant 31–32
  preovulatory 23–32
    LH importance for development
    75–81
follicular development 24, 49–64
  atresia 49, 54–63
  case studies 75–81
    efficacy study 106–107, 109
    first established pregnancy 70–71
    following multiple-dose
      administration 115–116,
      122–124, 126
    recombinant versus natural FSH
      158, 165–169
  estrogen role 126–127
  FSH role 18, 24, 49–64
  hCG supplementation effects
    49–50, 60–61
  LH role 18, 24, 49–64, 75–81
  two-cell two-gonadotropin theory
    4–5, 18, 50, 81
FSH *see* follicle stimulating hormone;
  recombinant FSH

gonadotropin-deficient subjects
  bioactivity following single recFSH
    injection 35–46
  multiple-dose administration
    115–127
gonadotropin-releasing hormone
  (GnRH)
  agonist regimens 99–110
granulosa cells
  FSH mechanism of action 4
  human granulosa cell cultures 25
  recFSH effects 23–32
    comparison with natural FSH
      26–28
    estradiol production 23, 26–32
    preovulatory follicles 28–30
    progesterone production 23,
      27–31
  regulation 81, 116

human chorionic gonadotropin
  (hCG) supplementation
  aromatase activity response 4, 13, 18
  follicular development and 49–50,
    63
  granulosa cell response and 26–27
  ovarian weight and 4, 13, 18, 60, 63
  plasma estradiol levels and 4, 13–16
  uterine weight and 60
  see also Pregnyl®
human menopausal gonadotropin
  (hMG) 4, 5, 158
hypogonadism 115–127
  male, spermatogenesis induction
    137–140
hypophysectomy 115, 117, 124

immunofluorometric assay 39
in vitro fertilization (IVF)
  first established pregnancy and
    birth using recFSH 69–73
  recFSH efficacy studies 99–110,
    143–154, 157–171
    cycle cancellations 168
    cycle outcome 108, 109
    embryo transfer 107–108
    oocyte retrieval 107–108
    ovarian stimulation 106–107
    pregnancy outcome 108
    safety aspects 109, 168
  recombinant versus natural FSH
    143–154, 157–171
inhibin serum levels
  case reports 70–71, 107, 109
  multiple-dose administration 116,
    120–124, 125, 127
isolated gonadotrophin deficiency
  75–81, 115, 117, 124

Kallman's syndrome 115, 117, 124

Leydig cell bioassay 4, 12–13, 17–18
LH *see* luteinizing hormone
LH surge 24, 28–32
luteinizing hormone (LH)
  estradiol levels and 15
  estrogen production and 75–81
  recFSH intrinsic LH activity 4, 12,
    14, 17–18, 127

role in follicular development 18, 24, 49–64, 75–81
serum levels 70–71, 152
  following multiple recFSH dose administration 115–116, 120–121
  following single recFSH injection 92–93

Metrodin® 143, 146, 157–171

oestradiol *see* estradiol
oestrogen synthesis *see* estrogen synthesis
oocyte retrieval
  efficacy study 100, 107–108, 109
  recombinant versus natural FSH 143, 150–151, 153, 157, 164–167, 169
Org 32489
  case studies
    bioactivity following single injection 35–46
    comparison with natural FSH 143–154, 157–171
    efficacy 99–110, 143–154, 157–171
    first established pregnancy and birth 69–73
    multiple-dose administration 115–127
    pregnancy and birth with polycystic ovary syndrome 131–134
    safety 85, 88, 90
    single-dose pharmacokinetics 85–96
    spermatogenesis induction 137–140
    tolerance 85, 90
  effects on granulosa cells 23–32
  see also recombinant FSH
ovarian hyperstimulation syndrome 153–154, 168, 170
ovarian stimulation
  efficacy study 106–107
  first established pregnancy and birth 69–73
  with polycystic ovary syndrome 131–134
  following multiple-dose administration 115–127
  recombinant versus natural FSH 143–154, 157–171
  see also follicular development
ovarian weight 4, 13–16, 49, 53–54
  effect of hCG supplementation 4, 13, 18, 49, 60, 63
  effects of recombinant versus natural FSH 15–16
  see also follicular development
ovulation induction *see* ovarian stimulation

panhypopituitarism 117
pharmacokinetics, single-dose 85–86, 90–96
pituitary FSH *see* follicle stimulating hormone
polycystic ovary syndrome 126
  first established pregnancy and birth 131–134
pregnancy
  efficacy study 100, 108–109
  recombinant versus natural FSH 143–144, 150–151, 157–158, 164–165, 170
  first case report 69–73
  with polycystic ovary syndrome 131–134
Pregnyl® 132, 139, 147
preovulatory follicles
  LH importance for development 75–81
  recFSH effects 23–32
primary efficacy parameters 151, 164–165
progesterone
  granulosa cell response 23, 27–31
  serum levels 70–72, 152
Puregon® *see* Org 32489

receptor displacement studies 7, 10, 12, 17
recombinant FSH (recFSH)
  absorption rate 45, 94–95
    sex differences 86, 94–95
  aromatase activity response 4, 13–18
  case studies
    absorption 86, 94–96

efficacy studies 99–110, 143–154, 157–171
first established pregnancy and birth 69–73
multiple-dose administration 115–127
pregnancy and birth with polycystic ovary syndrome 131–134
safety 85, 88, 90, 143–145, 153
single-dose pharmacokinetics 85–96
spermatogenesis induction 137–140
tolerance 85, 90
comparison with natural FSH 3–19
bioactivity following single injection 35–46
effects on granulosa cells 26–28
efficacy 143–154, 157–171
immunoreactivity following single injection 35–46
in vitro bioassay studies 3, 7–11, 17
in vitro neutralization of bioactivity 10, 13
receptor displacement studies 3, 7, 10, 12, 17
safety 143–154
follicular growth induction 18, 49–64, 75–81
granulosa cell responses 23–32
estradiol production 23, 26–32
preovulatory follicles 28–30
progesterone production 23, 27–31
hCG supplementation 4, 13–16, 18
follicular growth and 60–61, 63
intrinsic LH activity 4, 12, 14, 17–18, 127
ovarian weight response 4, 13–16, 49, 53–54
plasma estradiol response 4, 13–15, 53–54, 62
specific activities 17
testosterone production induction 4, 12, 14

safety 85, 90, 109
parameters 88, 160
recombinant versus natural FSH 143–145, 153, 168
secondary efficacy parameters 151, 165–167
serum levels
androstenedione 120–121, 125
estradiol 4, 13–16, 53–54, 62
hCG supplementation effects 4, 13–16
FSH 75, 79–80
body weight and 86, 92–93
efficacy study 106–107
first established pregnancy 70–71
following multiple-dose administration 115–116, 120–125
recombinant versus natural FSH 152, 165–166
single-dose pharmacokinetics 35–46, 86, 90–92
inhibin 70–71, 107, 116, 120–125, 127
LH 70–71, 152
following multiple recFSH dose administration 115–116, 120–121
following single recFSH injection 92–93
progesterone 70–72, 152
testosterone 120–124, 125
spermatogenesis induction 137–140

testosterone
induction by recFSH 4, 12, 14, 17–18
serum levels following recFSH injection 120–124, 125
tolerance 85, 90
triptorelin 99, 109, 145, 146
two-cell two-gonadotropin theory 4–5, 18, 50, 81

urinary FSH *see* follicle stimulating hormone
uterine weight 49, 53–54, 60, 62–64